The "3 Apple-a-Day" Plan

Your Foundation for Permanent Fat Loss

Tammi Flynn, M.S., R.D.
Jeanne Drury

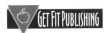

GET FIT PUBLISHING

Wenatchee, Washington

The "3 Apple-a-Day" Plan
Your Foundation for Permanent Fat Loss
By Tammi Flynn, M.S., R.D.

Published by:
Get Fit Publishing
P.O. Box 2226
Wenatchee, WA 98807-2226

www.3Appleplan.com

This book is not intended to replace the services of a physician or dietitian. Any application of the recommendations set forth in the following pages is at the reader's discretion. The reader should consult with his or her own physician or dietitian concerning the recommendations in this book.

Copyright © 2003 by Tammi Flynn

ISBN, print ed. 0-9745320-0-2

Printed in the United States of America

Library of Congress Cataloging-in-Publication Data

Edited and written in part by Jeanne Drury
Designed by Ken Trimpe
Food Photography by Rich Villacres
Food Styling by Cindy Marshall
Distributed by Get Fit Foods™

Table of Contents

PART I
THE "3 APPLE-A-DAY" PLAN

PART II
MENTAL PREPARATION

PART III
GOOD NUTRITION

PART IV
EXERCISE—A KEY TO STAYING YOUNG

PART V
SUCCESS STORIES

PART VI
MEAL PLANS AND RECIPES

PART VII

Dedication and Acknowledgments

This book is dedicated to my sisters, Tia and Teri, as well as those of you who are seeking balance and control over food and exercise issues. Finding the path of health that allows you to enjoy the process of eating healthy and exercising will provide you with a sense of well-being and peace—in mind, body and spirit.

All the best,
Tammi

My heartfelt thanks to my friends and family, who have supported me during my book-writing adventure. Cathy Covey, who gave me a copy of *Self Publishing Manual*, has kept me focused and encouraged through it all.

Others who have helped to assure accuracy, thoroughness, and creativity throughout the book—Jenny Hymer, Jacki Thomas, Blair McHaney, Chris Lyons, Alice Thompson, Jan Vetter and her daughter, Emma, Dr. Kolokoff, my editor, Jeanne Drury, and designer Ken Trimpe (for pulling those all-nighters!)

I especially thank my husband, Dan, who allowed me quiet time and took our three boys to the lake over the weekends. He's truly my best friend and partner, always providing the support and encouragement I need, whatever the endeavor may be.

Finally, many, many thanks to all of you who shared your photos, personal stories, quotes, and wonderful recipes. You made The "3 Apple-a-Day" Plan a success.

Thank you all!

"Just knowing what to do is not enough. You need confidence, motivation and a plan to make permanent changes."

- Anonymous

About the Author

Tammi Flynn is a registered dietitian who holds a Masters Degree in Nutrition Science from Texas A&M University, where she conducted her thesis on the effects of saturated and unsaturated fats on blood lipids. She is currently a group training instructor and staff dietitian at Gold's Gym in Wenatchee, Washington. She is also an accomplished body builder (2nd Place—2000 Team Universe, New York and 3rd Place—2000 USA Nationals, Las Vegas), an avid sports enthusiast (ice hockey, soccer, cycling and running) and a proud mother of three.

Tammi's educational background and interest in food and it's effect on health inspired her to open a successful low-fat bakery where she developed many recipes in this book. Her focus on healthy eating and physical fitness led not only to very effective weight loss programs at Gold's, but to the creation of the "3 Apple-a-Day" Plan, which she designed for a local contest.

The Plan came to national attention when 346 contestants, who lost a phenomenal 6,126 pounds of fat in just 12 weeks, attributed the apples in the Plan for the accelerated fat loss that the majority of them experienced. Many of their inspiring stories are in this book.

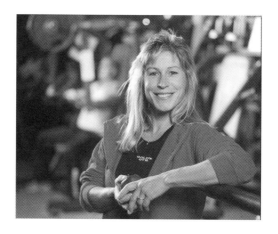

Getting Started

How much do you want to know?
1. Ready to start the plan today? Go to Quick Start on page 71.
2. Want to learn just the basics? Read only the Key Points at the end of each Part (I, II, III and IV).
3. Want to know the science behind the plan? Read from cover to cover!

Ideas to jumpstart your motivation
- Take pictures of yourself in a swimsuit (2-piece), front and back, and decide if you want to make a change.
- Train for a marathon.
- Take your doctor's advice to shape up.
- Train to climb Mt. Everest.
- Create a "get-fit" contest in your office.
- Train like an athlete.
- Enroll your family in a "Fit Family Group" and get healthy together.
- Buy an expensive swimsuit in a smaller size and plan a trip to Hawaii.
- Go to your 20-year reunion and check out an old flame or, better yet, the prom queen who snubbed you because you were fat!

Personal Contract

"Finding optimum health is a journey worth taking" - Anonymous

I,_____ plan to accomplish my ultimate goal of_____
_____. To reach this goal, I have established several mini goals
which are as follows: 1._____, 2._____,
3._____. I begin my journey on this date_____.
I would like to reach my ultimate goal by this date_____. If I don't,
I will continue to move forward and redefine my goals. My motivation level is
(circle one) high, very high, extremely high. As I reach each of my mini goals, I
will reward myself by_____

_____

Signed by_____
Date_____
Support person*_____

Check in with this person every two weeks and let them know how you are doing.

Introduction

The "3 Apple-a-Day" Plan is not about eating apples because they are healthy, even though it's a proven fact that they are. It's about shedding unhealthy fat layers, building strength, keeping lean muscle and transforming yourself—body and mind—into a fit, self-confident, full-of-life person.

The Plan came about by accident as part of the "Get-Lean" Diet I designed for a fitness contest at our gym. In an effort to include more fiber in the diet, in the form of fruits and vegetables, I added an apple before each meal. The results were absolutely astonishing! Who would have guessed that 346 people would lose 6,126 pounds of fat in 12 weeks? Since then, the "accident" has been repeated countless times from coast-to-coast—with the same amazing fat loss and body sculpting results. Read some of the personal success stories in Part V.

If you're tired of diets, pills and gimmicks, and tired of being a human garbage pail for all kinds of "convenience" foods (that are insidiously turning Americans into the fattest, unhealthiest people on earth) start the "3 Apple-a-Day" Plan today for good health, good nutrition, and *permanent fat loss.*

One more thing—be prepared to look and feel fabulous!

How and why it works

The "3 Apple-a-Day" Plan offers a variety of meals and over 100 recipes, custom designed to feed your muscle, not your fat. Each meal is calculated to provide your body with a balance of lean (low-fat) proteins, low-glycemic (based on the Glycemic Index, or GI), high fiber carbohydrates and essential fats. This balance will keep your blood sugar and insulin levels stable, which is necessary for your body to get into a "fat burning" mode. This balance also helps control your appetite, so you are less tempted by unhealthy foods. The calories, protein, carbohydrates and fat are all based on your current weight so you can maintain lean muscle tissue while shedding the fat.

The "3 Apple-a-Day" Plan, with its moderately high protein level, is similar to some of the popular high protein diets—at first glance. The level of protein provides calories that do not raise blood sugar, stabilizes blood sugar levels when eaten with carbohydrates, and provides necessary building blocks for maintaining muscle tissue.

Why it's different

This plan differs from those high protein diets in two major ways:

1. The focus of the "3 Apple-a-Day" Plan is not on weight loss alone, but primarily fat loss and muscle retention. Many popular diets are based

strictly on weight loss, regardless of whether the weight loss is from muscle tissue or fat. When muscle tissue is lost, our metabolism decreases, making it difficult for permanent weight loss.

2. Other high protein diets are very low in carbohydrates and high in fat, which induces ketosis (a high accumulation of ketones—see Chapter 7 for more on ketosis). People do lose weight quickly with those plans, but again, may lose valuable muscle tissue resulting in difficulty keeping the weight off. With low carbohydrate consumption comes some unpleasant side effects, too, such as constipation (due to lack of fiber or bulking carbohydrates), low energy or fatigue during exercise, not to mention mental confusion and moodiness! As if we aren't moody enough already!

In my professional experience, low carbohydrates and/or ketosis is not an optimum way to retain muscle tissue and achieve permanent fat loss. The key to carbohydrates is to consume enough for normal bodily functions (bowel elimination, fuel for the brain and red blood cells), but not in excess that may impede maximum fat loss.

In the following chapters, you'll find out how, by consuming proteins, carbohydrates, fats and fiber in the right combinations, you can be successful at permanent fat loss. You'll also find out why thousands of successful "losers" call the "3 Apple-a-Day" Plan the "terminator" of all diets!

PART I

The "3 Apple-a-Day" Plan

❖

The Creation of the "3 Apple-a-Day" Plan

Overweight vs. Overfat

Genetics and Obesity

❖

Chapter 1
The Creation of the "3 Apple-a-Day" Plan

The beginning

It all started when the American Cancer Society's daily recommendation of five to nine daily servings of fruits and vegetables (in general, a serving is one cup raw or one-half cup cooked) was proving difficult for one of my personal training clients. She was adamant about getting in her daily requirements, but struggling because she was extremely busy and traveled often. I asked her what her favorite fruit was and she said, "apples."

Perfect, I thought. Apples are full of important nutrients, have lots of fiber, taste delicious and, most important for her, they travel well. I suggested she eat an apple before each major meal (breakfast, lunch and dinner) to see if it would solve her problem.

Amazing results in just seven days

Just one week later, she came back to have her measurements (body composition test) redone saying since she'd been eating three apples a day, she felt her body had actually changed. She was excited because she hadn't made any changes for several months.

So we measured and, sure enough, she had lost one percent body fat in one week! Now, a one percent body fat loss (1.5 pounds of fat) in one week is difficult to accomplish in a fit person—and she was already lean at 16 percent body fat.

"Wow," I said, "Have you been running more?" She said the only thing she had done differently was to add apples to her meal plan (which actually increased her caloric intake!)

At this point, I was cautiously optimistic. I decided to try it on others to see if the results could be duplicated. When Gold's Gym of Wenatchee held their 12-week "Get-in-Shape" contest in January, 2001, I added apples to the diet (which was then called the "Get Lean" Diet).

The "Get-in-Shape" Contest

The annual 12-week contest, which I created in 1997, was (and is) a body transformation contest designed to lower body fat while retaining muscle tissue. Although judging is based primarily on visual change from before and after pictures, the body composition changes were also recorded. In this contest, we provided the diet, exercise recommendations, tips on calculating calories, protein, carbohydrates, fat, water and other information pertaining to the program.

Apples and the "Get Lean" Diet

The original "Get Lean" Diet was always a balance of low-glycemic (see Chapter 7 on glycemic response) carbohydrates, lean proteins, fruits and vegetables and essential fats—with a calorie distribution of 40 percent carbohydrates, 40 percent protein and 20 percent fat. On this balanced 12-week contest diet, women averaged five to seven percent body fat loss and men averaged seven to 10 percent loss.

In 2001, when apples were added to the "Get Lean" Diet, Gold's 12-week "Get-in-Shape" contest participants experienced record fat losses! Women averaged seven to 10 percent body fat losses and men averaged 10 to 12 percent losses. Not only that, two women broke the "most fat loss" record with 21 percent body fat loss each! One of those women, who later became a Gold's Gym National winner, lost a whopping 53 pounds of body fat and gained 10 pounds of muscle!

The following year, one male contestant lost 84 pounds of fat and acquired 19 pounds of lean muscle. Another man lost 85 pounds of fat and gained 26 pounds of lean, calorie-burning muscle (see Success Stories section).

Remember, these changes were made in just 12 weeks!

What a bunch of (happy) losers!

We were on a roll and truly excited with what we had accomplished. In the 2002 contest, 346 people lost 6,126 pounds of fat. In 2003, 351 people lost 6,453 pounds of fat! In both of those years *five of the 10* Gold's National contest winners hailed from Gold's Gym of little old Wenatchee, Washington!

What's the one thing Wenatchee winners all had in common? You guessed it…apples!

But was it *really* the apples?

After the first year of adding apples, even with all our contest successes, I still had reservations about whether apples were actually what helped these contestants lose more body fat than in past years. But adding apples was the only change we had made in the program.

Actually, I had eaten apples for many years when I was dieting for body building contests, but I never connected them with losing body fat. In fact, I kind of felt like I was cheating when I ate them during my contest dieting phase—because they tasted so good!

It wasn't until I had read some of the contestants' amazing and inspiring personal stories—a requirement for completion of the contest—that I was finally convinced. There were too many testimonials naming apples as a major contributor to their success to be a mere coincidence.

The $500,000 Gold's Gym Challenge

I became a true believer and I was not alone. The entire Gold's Gym staff was so strongly convinced that apples were a key to people's weight loss efforts that we approached the Washington Apple Commission and Gold's Gym Corporate about sponsoring a national contest.

Of course, they were skeptical at first. But with real numbers, testimonials and real contestants, they bought off on the idea and the $500,000 Gold's Gym Challenge was born. At the same time, Gold's Gym Corporate adopted the Washington apple as "The Official Diet Pill of Gold's Gym."

How and why do apples work in fat loss?

"I was never hungry. In fact, I had to retrain myself to eat enough. Never tiring of the three apples per day, I had no cravings for sweets. I believe the sweet Fuji apples helped in this area. I looked forward to having my apple as a snack every night! I had more energy, and was amazed at how steadily I lost weight. I plan to continue using the "3 Apple-a- Day" Plan to maintain my weight."

Sandi Anderson, age 53, lost 31 pounds of fat, gained two pounds of muscle in 12 weeks.

When the Challenge began, I started getting a lot of questions about apples, mostly wanting to know how they work in fat loss and what research I had to back up the claims.

Frankly, I was unaware of any research studies that linked apples to weight loss—let alone fat loss! Apples were chosen originally due to their convenience, sweet, crunchy texture and high fiber content (four to five grams per apple). I had found a few studies linking increased fiber intake to weight loss, by decreasing hunger and food intake, but none naming apples as the fiber source.

Recently, a Brazilian study of overweight women compared diets that contained either three apples per day, three pears per day or oat cookies, to determine their respective effects on body weight. The results showed the women who ate either three apples or three pears per day lost significantly more weight than the oat cookie group. This study is similar to what we found in our Gold's Gym contest.

In a more general sense, a 12-year Harvard study of 74,000 women concluded that those who consumed more fruits and vegetables were 26 percent less likely to become obese than women who ate fewer fruits and vegetables over the same time period.

Also, many studies have shown that apples can help in other aspects of health, such as heart disease and stroke prevention, improved lung function, dental health, and cancer prevention.

The phenomenal increase in fat loss when apples were added to diet plans of thousands of Gold's Gym clients, along with their personal testimonials naming apples as a key component to their success, is a more compelling reason for controlled studies to be done at the scientific level.

Right now, we'll settle for what works!

Good news for Type II Diabetics

The "3 Apple-a-Day" Plan is also used by Gold's Gym of Wenatchee in other challenges. One of those, the Type II Diabetes Challenge, is a six-month program based on a point system. Similar to the'"Get-in-Shape" contest using the same diet and measuring body fat only, the contestants were also required to keep food, beverage, medicine and exercise journals, have blood sugar checks twice daily, weekly blood pressure readings, pre and post lipid (blood fats) profiles, including cholesterol and triglycerides (see Chapter 10), and A1C (a measure used to determine long term blood sugar control). The participants did not have any kidney dysfunction prior to starting or finishing the challenge.

The results from that challenge showed the group that ate at least three apples per day lost an average of 19 pounds of body fat. The group that ate only one to two apples per day, lost 11 pounds of body fat. The other group that ate one or less apple per day, only lost three pounds of body fat. Overall, the average A1C reading was reduced from 7.5 starting to under five (normal range) at the finish.

Similar results were found with our six-month Wellness Challenge. The parameters were similar as far as keeping food, beverage, medicine and exercise journals, plus pre and post lipid and glucose panels. Again, the correlation to the three apples and greatest fat loss were observed, along with a total cholesterol (mainly LDL) lowering effect.

We have only suggested whole, fresh apples with the peels and have not compared them to peeled apples, apple juice, applesauce or dried apples. The apples, in conjunction with a balanced meal and exercise plan, have given many great results. These are only a few groups, however, and more controlled studies should be done to determine how apples may help with fat loss.

Worried about Cholesterol? More good news

Most people who had high blood lipids before following the plan experienced dramatic changes in their blood work afterwards. Exercise and eating the foods on the plan not only lowered their total cholesterol, LDL's, triglycerides and blood pressure, it increased their HDL's (good cholesterol).

Here's a great example. Byron, a 40 year-old male, started with an unhealthy cholesterol level of 211 and a triglyceride level of 637. In week 11 of the program, his cholesterol fell to an amazing 97 (low end of the range) and triglycerides to 51 (normal range)! On top of that, his HDL improved from a low of 25 to a normal level of 35. With astonishment, his physician asked if he felt okay and suggested they double check to make sure the reading was accurate. Byron said he hadn't felt this good since high school. And yes, the reading was accurate!

Others around the country also had improvements in their blood work. Richard from Utah lost 36 pounds and lowered his cholesterol from 218 to 152. More importantly, his LDL went from 128 to 86 and triglycerides from 270 to 61. His HDL increased from 36 to 49.

Scott from Maine lost 83 pounds and lowered his cholesterol from 243 to 125. His LDL dropped from 133 to 58, and his triglycerides went from 220 to 55.

Pete from Florida lost 53 pounds, lowered his cholesterol from 278 to 176, decreased LDL from 180 to 116 and triglycerides from 309 to 58. His HDL improved from 36 to 48. Pete's doctor told him he was a heartbeat away from a heart attack before he started the "3 Apple-a-Day" Plan. When his final blood work was done, the doctor couldn't believe the improvements he had made in just 12 weeks!

Who can use this Plan?

The "3 Apple-a-Day" Plan is useful for most people. My clients consist of females and males of all ages—ranging from 18 to 80—many of whom have adopted the plan for their entire family. Others, who have heart disease, high blood pressure, thyroid dysfunction, and Type II Diabetes, are interested in improving their health and reducing their medications.

As mentioned earlier, one group that has been very successful using this plan is Type II Diabetics. According to the Centers for Disease Control (CDC), there are 17 million Americans with Type II Diabetes, currently termed the "obese disease." This number has tripled since 1960 and is anticipated to triple again by 2050. By that time, one in three children born in 2000 will have diabetes if a healthier lifestyle isn't adopted—meaning healthier eating and exercise. What's even more frightening, the CDC estimates 70 million Americans are currently overweight, including one out of four children!

What exactly do we mean by "overweight?" That's a tricky question, which I'll discuss in the next chapter. The answer may surprise you!

Always check with your physician before starting a food program, especially if you have had previous health risks.

Chapter 2
Overweight vs. Overfat

What's the difference?

Researchers have learned that body fat, rather than weight, is a better predictor of health. High body fat, or overfat, is associated with diseases such as Type II Diabetes, heart disease, high blood pressure, insulin resistance and cancer, to name a few.

Being overfat is more dangerous to your health than being overweight. Traditionally, overweight has been defined as weighing more than the healthy weight listed for your age and height in a weight table. But that doesn't account for differences in body composition. For example, athletes are often overweight by the weight-table standards because of muscle development or large body frame, but are probably not overfat.

The "3 Apple-a-Day" Plan was specifically designed and developed for permanent fat loss and muscle retention (keeping lean muscle tissue). This Plan was not necessarily designed for weight loss—at least using the traditional method of measure (the scale). Other measuring techniques to determine progress have been highly effective and motivational. These include girth measurements (waist, hip, and thigh), body composition testing and body mass index (BMI), which we'll get into later.

The scale only tells you the partial truth!

Weighing yourself on a bathroom scale tells you next to nothing about how healthy you really are. Gaining or losing a pound doesn't always mean it's a pound of fat. In fact, small frequent shifts in weight typically reflect fluid changes in your body. Your body's fluid levels vary depending on the amount of salt you eat, your activity level and your hormone changes. It seems that many people, mainly women, are controlled by the numbers on the scale. If the number goes up, they're discouraged. If the number goes down, they are motivated and happy. The numbers on the scale do not measure the progress you have made and can be detrimental to your program. *Why not break those barriers and get permanent results without the frustration of the scale?* The following chart shows how different body types and body fat levels can all be at the same body weight.

Males 40-49 years old

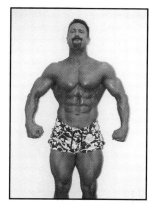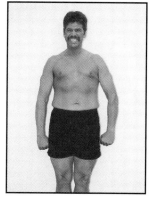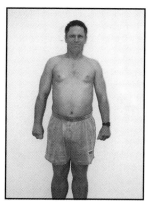

Body Fat: 5 %   15.5 %   26 %

These men all weigh 195 pounds!

Females 30-39 years old

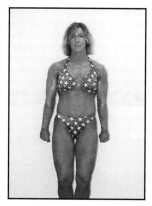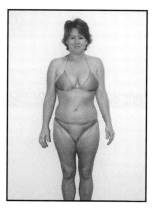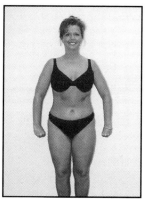

Body Fat: 13 %   23 %   31 %

These women all weigh 135 pounds!

Get the picture?

Other methods for measuring

Methods of body fat measuring, which can be determined by a trained professional, are skinfold measurements, infrared interactance, bioelectrical impedance or underwater weighing. Other methods, such as girth measurements and BMI, can be done at home. A BMI reading is just a gauge in determining health risk. This measurement may not be appropriate for athletes or very active people.

For girth measurements, use a tape measure around the waist at the navel, measure hips around the buttocks and measure the upper part of the thigh. For every one inch lost from the waist is equal to 4 pounds of body fat (*Muscle and Fitness* magazine, March, 2003).

To determine BMI, calculate from the following formula:

Weight (pounds) ÷ Height (inches)^2 x 703 = BMI

Example: Female, 5 foot 4 inches, 140 pounds
140 ÷ (64" x 64") x 703 = 24

Male, 5 foot 11 inches, 185 pounds
185 ÷ (71" x 71") x 703 = 25.79

If your BMI ranges from 18.5 to 24.9, your weight is not likely to have a major effect on your health. If your BMI is 25 or more, talk to your physician about the "3 Apple-a-Day" Plan.

Is your health at risk?

- Do you eat at *least* five servings of fruits and vegetables per day?
- Are you physically active at least 30 minutes per day, seven days per week?
- Do you eat less than three deep fried foods per week?
- Is your waist measurement under 35 inches for a female? Under 40 inches for a male?
- Is your BMI under 25?
- Do you consider yourself at a healthy body fat level?
- Does your family history show healthy body weights without obesity?

If you can answer yes to most of these questions, you're probably not at a high risk of developing overfat related diseases. If you answered no to at least three of the questions, your chances are greater for developing overfat related diseases.

This is not a medically proven questionnaire to determine the risk of becoming overfat. It is exclusively used as a screening technique for increasing health awareness.

Chapter 3
Genetics and Obesity

Were we born to be fat?

Genetics play a role in your body type and how you store fat. However, other factors greatly influence your risk of being fat or overfat—factors that you can change or prevent.

The big fat facts of life

Fact one: you can't always blame your parents. Yes, a family history of obesity does increase your chances of becoming obese (overfat) by about 30 percent, as well as your eating habits and activity levels as a child. But the other 70 percent is influenced by what you do now, as an adult. Your genes affect the rate at which your body accumulates fat and where the fat is stored. You are born with a predetermined amount of fat cells—that can't be changed without surgery.

Fact two: unfortunately, you have an unlimited amount of potential fat cells leading to obesity and obesity related diseases if overeating and under exercising continues.

So now's the time to start making changes.

The difference between boys and girls

Have you ever wondered why men seem to lose weight at the drop of a hat, and women seem to have more of a struggle? Or why building muscle seems to come naturally to guys but takes longer for us gals? Does "you are what you eat" ring a bell?

In my 20 years of experience in the health and fitness industry, I have observed that men and women have different preferences, which may influence how they lose body fat. When it comes to food preferences, for example, males tend to choose protein over carbohydrates. With physical preferences, they go for the weight training every time—with as little cardiovascular training as possible.

Females, on the other hand, prefer carbohydrates over protein for their food choices, and choose walking for weight loss (cardiovascular training) instead of weight training.

Are you connecting the dots?

Muscle, fat and metabolism

Due to their higher muscle mass, males tend to burn 10-20 percent more calories than females (who have higher body fat levels). Think about this: one pound of muscle tissue burns 40-60 calories per day whereas one pound of fat tissue burns a measly two calories per day. No wonder these guys lose weight so easily! Their higher muscle mass endows them with a higher metabolic rate. But ladies, you can change all that by adding some muscle mass through weight training!

Use it or lose it!

As you age, if you do not use your muscles, you'll lose them (the muscle tissue shrinks), thus resulting in lower metabolism and an inability to burn calories. Starting around age 25, you lose about one percent of muscle every year, which results in a reduction of metabolism. So let's do the math.

By the age of 35, you would lose approximately five pounds of muscle. For each pound of muscle lost, you'll lose the ability to burn the 40-60 calories per day. So five pounds (muscle) x 40-60 calories equals 200-300 calories less that your body could burn per day! By the age of 50, you may have lost 25 pounds of muscle, reducing your calorie burning ability by 1000 calories. You begin to notice that you eat less, but you are getting fatter! Although this may be some-what exaggerated, I think you get the point.

But all is not lost. Weight training increases muscle mass, which increases your ability to burn calories. It's possible to minimize, even reverse some of the damage from inactivity—if you start now!

If your goal is permanent fat loss, weight training is the answer (see Part IV on Exercise).

Key Points from Part I

- Try to see the big picture. Having a balanced meal and exercise plan results in giving you a sense of control and peace in your journey.
- The "3 Apple-a-Day" Plan is a balance of lean proteins, low-glycemic, high-fiber carbohydrates and essential fats.
- Eat three apples per day, one before each major meal.
- Apples are full of fiber—four to five grams each.
- Fiber has been shown to be effective in weight loss.
- Being overfat, not just overweight, has a higher risk factor for obesity-related diseases.
- Avoid the scale for measuring your fitness progress. Use other methods.
- Use the BMI to determine your health risk.
- Genetics has only a small influence on becoming overfat. You have 70 percent control.
- Muscle tissue burns more calories than fat tissue.
- Weight training builds muscle tissue.

PART II

Mental Preparation

You Have the Power

The Importance of Setting Goals

Chapter 4
You Have the Power!

If your eating habits have been less than healthy, you have the power to make the change! Every step you take to improve your health will get you closer to adding life to your years. The foods you choose, along with your activity level, will determine whether you become fat or not. The most notable causes of being overfat or obese are lack of proper diet and physical activity. Thank goodness, those are things you can change. If you can visualize it, you can become it!

"Being an obese, out-of-control Type II Diabetic, I talked with my physician, who said he could no longer help me, I had to help myself. Then I heard the words, "train like an athlete." So I started practicing being an athlete—started a food and exercise journal, joined the gym, bought athletic clothes so I could look like an athlete, and after work and days off I would change into my athletic clothes to feel like an athlete. So who cares if I looked like the Pillsbury Doughboy™, in my mind I was an athlete."

Donald Housden lost 33 pounds and now is an athlete.

Getting and staying motivated

How do you get motivated and stay motivated? Motivation comes from within. Webster's defines motivation as "a mental force to induce an act or purpose." Inspiration is any influence that inspires thought or action. What inspires you?

I have found that people are inspired by money, other people's successes and family. In the beginning, you may be motivated to win (through a bet), look like someone else (if they can do it, so can I), or believe if you can make a change, it will help inspire your family to change. But what will really keep you progressing towards your goal is how good you'll feel from your behavior changes. Some people are self-motivated and others need a little extra help from outside influences.

Tip: *Find something or someone that inspires you. Health Clubs can be inspirational because you're surrounded by people with a common interest—getting healthy!*

Are timelines a good thing?

Does focusing on a short period of time such, as 12-weeks versus a lifetime, prove unsuccessful for permanent fat loss? It all depends on whether you are enjoying the experience of getting fit or struggling throughout the entire process. You may be highly motivated when you first start a new diet or exercise program. However, motivation dissipates over time if you cannot see or feel results.

Most people who start the "3 Apple-a-Day" Plan adjust over the first few weeks. For some, it's more difficult—especially if they've never exercised or been aware of their eating habits. On the other hand, people who finish the 12 weeks are thrilled with their progress. And more importantly, most of them maintain their results.

Twelve weeks will pass by anyway, so why not do something during that time that will make a difference in how you look and feel? Think of 12 weeks as just the beginning of a lifetime of healthy behaviors.

> ***Tip:*** *Make small, realistic, short-term goals, which will lead you to your major goal. If you bite off more than you can chew, it can be overwhelming!*

One diet fits all—not!

The "one diet fits all" approach is not appropriate. Body types vary, which determines how people store fat. There are a variety of diets for various conditions. Diets should be tailored to the individual and reflect their specific purpose or goals. The "3 Apple-a-Day" Plan is designed for permanent fat loss and muscle retention. This plan is for people who want to look and feel better forever! The apples not only make this plan convenient, they provide fiber, help with hunger control and satisfy sweet cravings. On this plan, weight loss will occur gradually (the healthy way) and losing inches will occur more rapidly.

Although muscle is heavier than fat, it also takes up less space, so as your body fat comes down, your muscle will become more defined. The "3 Apple-a-Day" Plan has been used with various groups of males and females, ages 18 to 80 years old, some of which include elite and recreational athletes, sedentary and overweight people, Type II Diabetics and people with heart disease, high cholesterol, high blood pressure and arthritic conditions. Most have been successful at improving their conditions simply by making food and exercise changes.

> ***Tip:*** *A healthy program should consist of meal plans that include a balance of the basic food groups and an exercise program that includes muscle strengthening and cardiovascular training. To get started, add two or three apples to your current diet and start walking daily.*

Chapter 5

The Importance of Setting Goals

Health vs. fitness

Is your goal to improve your health or to improve your fitness? This is an important question to answer in order to determine what goals to set. Health improvement can be achieved by making simple or major changes such as: adding or increasing activity, improving diet, quitting smoking, reducing stress, getting adequate rest and laughing.

Yes, laughing. According to William Fry, M.D., Professor at Stanford University with 50 years of laughter research, laughter conditions the heart muscle, exercises the lungs, works all the abdominal thoracic muscles, boosts the immune system and even increases the adrenaline and blood flow to the brain. Humor can add years to your life! Many of these changes will reflect an improved mental health status, but not necessarily a noticeable physical change.

Fitness improvements may take more effort. But the resulting change in body fat, increased muscle tissue, cardiovascular and respiratory efficiency, and improved mental alertness will all be worth the extra sweat!

That said, fitness improvements require fitness-oriented goals including a regular exercise routine, a well-balanced meal plan, adequate rest and a plan of action. The "3 Apple-a-Day" Plan is designed for fitness oriented people, but most people can use this plan for health improvements, too.

Determining your goals

Do you want to run to your goal or walk? In other words, do you want to achieve your goal quickly or make gradual changes? Goals need to be set according to what you are planning to accomplish. The "3 Apple-a-Day" Plan was designed for people who want to lose body fat and keep their muscle tissue. The following examples may give you some ideas and guidance for other goals:

1. Although weight loss should not be the primary focus, most health experts agree that one or two pounds of weight loss per week is safe and healthy. Rapid and extreme weight loss can also result in muscle loss, which is often associated with low-calorie meal plans.

2. Reducing your clothes size is a measurable goal. Take out your smallest clothes size so they're visible. If you can see it, you can achieve it!

3. Waist, hip and thigh reduction—measure those areas and try to lose one

inch per month on your "problem" areas (waist or hips).

4. Lower your cholesterol, blood pressure or blood sugar by starting a regular exercise routine.

5. Increase your daily energy by improved eating habits and exercise. You can measure this by keeping a food and exercise journal (see journaling in this chapter).

6. Gain strength or increase lean muscle tissue through weight training. Improvements can be measured by increased weights lifted or body composition testing.

7. Commit to eating breakfast every day.

8. Switch the nightly food binge to fruits, vegetables or lean proteins only.

9. Reduce body fat to the healthy range—women 17-24 percent, men 14-20 percent.

10. Exercise for 20 minutes during the lunch hour daily.

The list can go on. It may take several small goals to achieve your results.

Tips from Gold's Gym past contest winners:

1. *Keep a food and exercise journal. This keeps you accountable and on track.*
2. *Focus on a specific goal. **Visualize your end result.** Keep reminding yourself that you are committed to achieving that goal.*
3. *Plan, prepare and commit.*

***Plan**—what you want to accomplish (goal), how long it will take you (timeline), how you can accomplish it (specific program).*

***Prepare**—know what you'll be eating and when you'll be exercising daily. Prepare meals ahead of time and plan your workout before you get to the gym.*

***Commit**—make a contract with yourself, spouse, children or trainer to accomplish your goals. Again, be specific and use this contract to hold yourself accountable.*

"If you fail to plan, you plan to fail." - Nancy Vanhoven,
Group fitness instructor,
Gold's Gym of Wenatchee, WA

Journaling prevents "amnesia"

Keeping a food and exercise journal is a key factor for maintaining weight loss. Writing down your accurate intake of food and beverages daily and recording the calories, protein, fat, carbohydrates and fiber will help you become more aware of what is in the foods you eat.

Writing it down will also hold you accountable for what you have been eating or drinking. Although you may have good intentions, what you intend and what you actually do may be two different things (amnesia). An exercise journal works the same way. You'll know if you are making progress by keeping records of where you were when you started. In the Appendix, you'll find a sample page for keeping a food and beverage journal.

Don't kid yourself

A frustrated client e-mailed me saying she had been following the Plan, but wasn't making any progress. I asked if she was writing it down. She wasn't. I asked her to keep a journal and send it to me after a few days, so I could see where she might be struggling. No wonder she hadn't made progress! Her journal indicated that she ate almost everything out of a box or container! Except for two apples per day she wasn't following the Plan at all. In addition, she hadn't changed her exercise program (walking) for over one year. I made some suggestions in order to accommodate her busy schedule (the reason for her dependence on convenience foods) and food preferences. A few weeks later, she e-mailed to say, happily I might add, she had finally started seeing some results.

Again, intentions are good, but writing it down is the only way to outsmart your biased and forgetful mind!

Breaking barriers and excuses, excuses, excuses!

Why is it that when we start an exercise or food program we often don't follow through? (As in "it seemed like a good idea at the time.") There are a few legitimate reasons (out of your control) that inhibit you from reaching your goals—such as illness or certain disabilities. But mostly, barriers may be excuses that keep you in your comfort zone—or rather, out of your discomfort zone! Changing eating and exercise habits may be one of the most difficult challenges you'll experience. But remember, the rewards you'll gain far outweigh those initial struggles.

Here are some of the common controllable barriers that factor into changing your lifestyle habits.

- *Not enough time to exercise.* Exercise needs to be a priority just like brushing your teeth!
- *You are confused about choice of programs.* Pick a program that includes all food groups and is appealing to your food preferences.
- *Too intimidated to go to the gym because you're out of shape.* Start walking or working out at home with exercise videos. But a good gym can offer professional help to guide you to your goals.
- *Belief that you need to eat very low calories to lose.* Eating too little calories is a sure bet to losing valuable muscle tissue. Women need at least 1200 calories per day, and men need at least 1800.
- *Environment.* You're surrounded by a feasting society. Fast foods and quick food markets are loaded with high fat, high sugar, nutrient-dense temptations. When you use discipline to plan and prepare your meals, the temptations will become less and you will not have to rely on willpower.
- *No energy or too tired.* You will get more energy by balancing your meal plan and exercising.

Beware of emotional triggers—they make you eat!

Have you ever been sad and sat down with a tub of ice cream smothered in chocolate and just kept eating it? Or been stressed out and stuffed a whole bag of chips (family size!) in your face? Or just felt bored and wandered through your kitchen "searching" for something interesting to eat, and discovered (and ate) your kid's leftover Halloween candy? Or felt the "wind down" of a busy day and needed a little "pick-me-up" from food?

This is called emotional eating. There are several emotional triggers—anger, stress/anxiety, PMS, boredom and sadness—that cause us to eat. And we usually don't choose healthy snacks in this state of mind. Instead, we choose "comfort foods" that temporarily fill the void. Often, we not only consume way too much of these foods, we repeat this type of eating way too often, all of which leads to weight gain and low self-esteem.

How to break the cycle

Breaking the cycle of emotional eating may take some effort. But you can do it! When you feel one or more of these emotions come on, resist the urge for five minutes. Ask yourself if you are truly hungry or just feeling emotional? Often just waiting a couple of minutes will be sufficient to overcome the urge. If not, and you are still feeling emotional, try diverting yourself. Go outside for some fresh air, take a walk, turn on some upbeat music, or call a supportive friend.

If you do decide to eat, choose a healthy snack. Dip some unsalted pretzels in yogurt or spread apple slices with peanut butter. Or treat yourself to some low-fat popcorn and a diet beverage. And don't turn on the television! Huh? That's right! Watching TV could actually cause you to "unconsciously" eat more.

I definitely have times of emotional overeating—where do you think the examples came from?! What I have found to work, besides avoiding unhealthy snacks, is having an established eating plan. When you follow the "3 Apple-a-Day" Plan, as I do, it will help keep your appetite under control and lessen those unhealthy food temptations.

Discipline vs. willpower

"If you have the discipline you will not need to rely on willpower," says Blair McHaney, Co-owner of Gold's Gym, Wenatchee, Washington. Discipline, according to Webster's Dictionary, is "mental and moral training; obedience to rules; a set of regulations; regimen." Willpower is defined as, "strength of will; self-discipline."

If you have a plan and you mentally prepare to fulfill the plan, you will not have to rely on willpower. It is only when you feel weak or vulnerable that food temptations will test your willpower—if you aren't self-disciplined.

> ***Tip:*** *Plan and prepare your food and exercise regimen ahead of time. Make the commitment to yourself to carry out your plan.*

Hunger vs. appetite

Blair McHaney also suggests this visual. "Think of appetite as a sleeping lion. If you keep him fed, he will purr and sleep. If you starve him, he will attack." The attack is your appetite. If you aren't prepared with food on hand, your appetite may take over and you'll be relying on your willpower. That's doing it the hard way for sure.

It's a lot easier to shop for healthy foods in the grocery store if you are not hungry as a lion going in. Not only that, you'll be less likely to buy unhealthy items. It's much easier to decide not to buy "junk" food than it is to resist it once you've taken it home. Keep your home environment safe and junk-food-free to avoid temptation.

Last but not least, eat breakfast! You'll be less likely to eat a donut at work.

> ***Tip:*** *Take apples with you everywhere you go.*

Key Points of Part II

- If you can visualize what you want to become, it will happen.
- Find a food and exercise program that is conducive to your goals and keep a journal.
- Set your ultimate goal. Make sure it's realistic and measurable.
- Set mini goals that are measurable to reach your ultimate goal.
- Find inspiration to motivate you.
- Decide on health or fitness goals.
- Break the barriers that prevent you from reaching your goal.
- Discipline yourself by preparing and planning so willpower won't be an issue.

PART III

Good Nutrition

❖

The Truth About Nutrition, Diet and Fat Loss

Carbohydrates—Good Food for Your Brain

Protein—The Body's Building Blocks

Fats—Healthy vs. Unhealthy

Cholesterol and Triglycerides

Energy, Water and Alcohol

Metabolic Cost of Food and Meal Frequency

Dining Out, Portion Control, Convenience and Supplements

❖

*Note: The content in this section is important to know,
but not necessary to succeed with this plan.
If you would like to know the details on how
carbohydrates, protein and fat function,
read this section. If not, skip to Chapter 11.*

Chapter 6
The Truth about Nutrition, Diet and Fat Loss

Mass confusion

There are simply too many diet books, versions of food pyramids, guidelines and other nutritional advice on the market today. Each one would have you believe theirs is *the one*. Much of the information is conflicting. Should you eat low-fat, high carbohydrates? Or low-carbohydrate, high fat? Should you eat high protein, high fat? How about the no dairy, no wheat, no fat, no meat (and no flavor) diet? Just kidding!

Amid the cacophony of opinions, there is one thing that most experts do agree on. Most people are overfat due to lack of fruit and vegetable intake and physical activity. It's as simple as that.

The low calorie weight loss trap

"I laughed when I heard the phrase, "skinny fat person," and then it hit me. That's what I have ended up being every time I went on a diet because all that I did was stop eating and didn't have a real exercise program. Then my weight always ended up coming back even heavier than I was to begin with!"

**Jim Barker, age 51, lost 43.5 pounds of body fat
and gained 0.5 pounds of muscle.**

Many of the popular programs these days are based strictly on weight loss, which can be beneficial for many reasons aside from appearance—*but only if you can maintain your current muscle mass.*

Some of these plans are downright harmful, especially if permanent fat loss is your goal. For example, the diets based on very low calories are the biggest trap of all! They are seductive in that they offer quick results. But in the long term they are disastrous. Ultra-low-calorie diets are the cause of yo-yo dieting, which lowers your metabolism incrementally over time until it's almost impossible to lose weight.

Research from the University of California has shown that crash diets—of less than 1,000 calories a day—slows metabolism down by as much as 45 percent!

These diets fly in the face of what is now common knowledge: to raise your metabolism, you have to *eat more healthy foods, not less*! Eating less lowers your metabolism by stripping away your muscle tissue and is the direct cause of plateaus that are so hard to overcome. It's likely you'll become a "skinny fat person" if you follow a low-calorie eating program.

"But," you reason, "if I eat more I'll just gain weight." I reply, "Not if you eat healthy foods and exercise you won't!" If you consume small, nutritionally balanced, low glycemic meals, at regular intervals throughout the day, your metabolism will be revved up all day long!

In other words, the "3 Apple-a-Day" Plan.

Why I wrote this book

I'm not a diet guru on the talk show circuit, I'm not selling supplements or magic weight loss powders. What I am is a registered dietitian, a body-builder and a group training instructor with 20 years of experience in helping my clients lose fat, get fit—and stay fit.

My purpose in writing this book is to use my knowledge of nutrition, diet and exercise to guide you to *permanent fat loss and muscle retention* without diet pills, supplements or gimmicks. I would also like to clear the air of the confusion and disinformation associated with nutrition and weight loss. And share many of our success stories.

The "3 Apple-a-Day" Plan, which I developed for the Gold's Gym "Get-in-Shape" contest, uses all food groups in balanced proportions to help your metabolism do its job. It features apples due to their convenience, low glycemic rating and high fiber content—the latter two of which are extremely important in fat loss.

The control you need to succeed

The "3 Apple-a-Day" Plan will give you the control you must have over your appetite in order to achieve your weight loss goals—by balancing carbohydrates, proteins and essential fats.

It's for people who want to make the most out of their lives, without perpetually looking for the one and only "next best diet." Most importantly, this plan has been successful in helping people achieve *permanent* fat loss when combined with an exercise plan.

New recommendations

As of September 5, 2003, the Institute of Medicine's Food and Nutrition Board released it's revised reports of Dietary Reference Intakes (DRI's) for energy, carbohydrates, fiber, fat, fatty acids, protein (known collectively as macronutrients) and exercise. Each will be discussed in appropriate chapters and referred to as the DRI's.

Chapter 7

Carbohydrates—Good Food For Your Brain

The misunderstood nutrient

I feel good when I think of carbohydrates, because I know they provide the right kind of fuel for my brain cells. Unfortunately, many people shun them as if they were the plague. The fact is, carbohydrates have gotten a bad rap recently for weight loss efforts, just like fat has in years past.

What's more, (and what many dieters aren't aware of) the types of carbohydrates you choose can affect your fat loss progress to a *very high degree*. So let's set the record straight with the facts on carbohydrates.

Not all carbohydrates were created equal

Diet fads seem to come in cycles. Remember when protein was the enemy and carbohydrates were "the answer?" Now the opposite philosophy is the "new big thing." However, with new findings about lean proteins, along with the Glycemic Index, it seems that we were only half right on both counts.

The role of carbohydrates

At any given moment the amount of carbohydrate in the adult body is about 300 grams or less. Some of this is in the blood, but most is stored in the liver and muscles as glycogen.

Carbohydrates have many functions, the chief of which is to provide, 1) energy to carry on the work of the body and, 2) heat to maintain the body's temperature. Glucose, which is the breakdown from carbohydrates, is the only form of energy used by the central nervous system, even though other tissues also use fats for energy.

Other things carbohydrates do

1. Carbohydrates spare proteins. This means that the body need not burn protein from the diet or body tissue to meet energy needs.
2. Carbohydrates aid in the manufacture of nonessential amino acids (refer to Chapter 8 on Protein).
3. Carbohydrate is required for the complete oxidation of fats. When too little carbohydrate is available, some fatty acids known as ketones accumulate. A high accumulation of ketones is called ketosis, which interferes with acid/base balance and causes the blood to become more acidic. Known as ketoacidosis, this condition can cause brain damage and eventually death. Dehydration is also a common consequence of

ketosis because the body loses water-excreting ketones in the urine.

All carbohydrates except fiber have four calories per gram. Fiber is not utilized for energy, therefore, does not have a caloric value.

Is your glycemic response making you fat?

Equal amounts of carbohydrates from a variety of foods such as sugar, pastas, legumes and breads can produce varying increases in blood glucose (blood sugar) in a given time. The immediate effect on blood glucose is ranked on the Glycemic Index (GI). As blood glucose levels rise, so does insulin, a hormone which helps shuttle blood glucose out of the blood into the cell to be used for energy. Insulin promotes fat storage.

High insulin levels are associated with obesity.

Choosing carbohydrates wisely

Carbohydrates are an essential part of a healthy meal plan. However, the amount and type of carbohydrate (in accordance to the Glycemic Index) will affect your fat loss efforts.

The fact is, the modern diet is too rich in high glycemic carbohydrates. Common high glycemic foods are cookies, crackers, bakery items, candy, snack items, simple sugars—some even claiming to be low-fat or healthy! This is one of the major reasons why Americans are getting fatter and fatter, with Type II Diabetes now showing up even in children who will, in turn, become the nation's next generation of even fatter adults.

Now is the time for high-profile nutritional education if we are to prevent a future health catastrophe.

It's never too late

It's never too late to change unhealthy habits. For example, middle-aged people accustomed to diets of high GI foods, can switch to low GI foods and be far less likely to develop diabetes and heart disease.

Low GI diets can also help control established diabetes by keeping blood glucose levels down. Low GI diets can also help you lose weight, may lower blood lipids, improve the body's sensitivity to insulin, reduce the Glycemic Index of the overall meal and improve appetite control.

Additionally, low GI carbohydrates satisfy your appetite without "over-satisfy-ing" your calorie requirement. This is discussed in detail in the *New Glucose Revolution*, a widely acclaimed book on the detrimental effects of high GI foods.

Examples of low glycemic foods are fruits (apples, cherries and pears), dairy products, stone-ground or whole grain products (oatmeal, brown rice, bulgar, some cereals and breads), beans and lentils.

In the "3 Apple-a-Day" Plan Substitution List (see Part VI), you'll find most carbohydrate foods have a glycemic rating. The following are the categories of low, intermediate and high glycemic rating of foods:

Low glycemic........below 55
Intermediate.........between 55-70
High glycemic.......more than 70

Protein (meats, fish and poultry) and fat (oils, nuts, and seeds) have little to no effect on glycemic response, therefore they play a vital role in keeping the glycemic response of a high GI food to a minimum. In other words, you won't get hungry an hour later.

The vicious cycle of high GI foods

High glycemic foods are effective in rapidly replenishing glycogen stores in endurance athletes. Unfortunately for regular, non-athletes, these foods tend to come from simple carbohydrates, such as sugar, which add empty calories.

Kathleen DesMaisons, PhD, author of *Potatoes not Prozac* concludes that many people who suffer from sugar sensitivity have a tendency to consume large quantities of sweets, breads, pasta or alcohol. Even though these items can trigger feelings of exhaustion and low self-esteem, their biochemical impact causes sugar-sensitive people to crave them even more.

This seemingly endless cycle can continue for years, leaving sufferers over-weight, fatigued, depressed and sometimes alcoholics.

The "3 Apple-a-Day" Plan is right on track

The primary carbohydrates in the "3 Apple-a-Day" Plan are from low-glycemic and high fiber sources. However, there are some intermediate and high-glycemic sources included in some of the recipes. According to the *Glucose Revolution* book, mixing a high glycemic food with a low glycemic food equals an intermediate glycemic meal.

Carbohydrate recommendations

The recommended DRI's, for both children and adults, are at least 130 grams of carbohydrates per day, based on the minimum needed to produce enough glucose for the brain to function.

The carbohydrate recommendation in the "3 Apple-a-Day" Plan is 40 percent of total calories (which is one gram per pound body weight). Carbohydrates in the Plan range from 128-187 grams per day (see Nutrient Chart in Chapter 11).

Tip: When you eat carbohydrates, other than what is listed on the Plan, choose those that have two to four grams of fiber per 100 calories. Whole grains, fruit and vegetables are good sources of fiber.

Fiber. It does more than keep you regular!

"Roughage" or "bulk" has been recommended for years for maintaining bowel regularity. Scientists and clinicians have found dietary fiber may reduce the risks of certain gastrointestinal diseases, diabetes, obesity, cardiovascular diseases, and possibly colon or rectal cancers.

Dietary fiber is an edible, non-digestible component of carbohydrates naturally found in plant food.

Two types of fiber

There are two general types of fiber: soluble and insoluble. Soluble fiber, such as oats and grains, may help reduce the risk of heart disease. Insoluble fiber, such as wheat, fruits and vegetables, is essential for healthy digestion and may reduce the risk of gastrointestinal diseases.

Unlike most fruits, apples have high amounts of both soluble and insoluble fiber. So, you're not only getting a heart healthy benefit, but a gut healthy one, too!

Modern diets are lacking in fiber due to the highly processed, conveniently available foods. The typical American diets that I have analyzed from seven-day food records averaged 10-13 grams of fiber per day. That is only one-third of both the DRI and American Cancer Society recommendations! Adding three apples per day will give you half of your fiber recommendation. Just add two or three servings of vegetables along with the apples and your fiber requirement is met for the day!

Fiber recommendations

The recommended DRI's for fiber range from 21-38 grams for adults, depending on age and gender. Fiber in the "3 Apple-a-Day" Plan ranges from 22-69 grams, depending on your calorie level (see Nutrient Chart in Chapter 11).

> ***Tip:*** *Adding too much fiber too fast can cause bloating, gas and cramps. If your diet has been low in fiber, gradually add the recommendations of fiber over several weeks to avoid discomfort.*

Chapter 8
Protein—The Body's Building Blocks

The great protein debate

Nutrition experts have long debated the ideal combination of proteins, carbohydrates and fats in respect to weight loss. Now with the return of the high protein diets, protein consumption is once again being debated, along with the conventional concerns related to saturated fats and cholesterol (see Chapter 9 on Fats).

Do moderately high protein diets that are low in saturated fats and cholesterol (like the "3 Apple-a-Day" Plan) raise the same concerns?

Study confirms the "3 Apple-a-Day" Plan basics

A 10-week study, led by Donald K. Layman, nutrition professor at the University of Illinois, found that women who ate 1700 calories, with protein based on body weight (0.73 grams of protein per pound body weight) lost body fat, maintained muscle and had improvement in total blood cholesterol. This group also reported to be less hungry between meals, experienced stable blood glucose levels and reduced insulin response following meals.

By comparison, participants in the study's control group consumed half as much protein of (0.36 grams per pound body weight), lost significantly less body fat and were unable to maintain muscle mass.

Dr. Katz, M.D., author of *The Way to Eat*, confirms that eating enough protein maximizes calorie-burning throughout the day. Research suggests that women who add two ounces of protein to each meal burn an extra 200 calories per day.

These studies confirm what I have found with various programs using the "3 Apple-a-Day" Plan. My clients who consume 40 percent of their calories from lean protein, report they are *less hungry between meals and have more control over their appetites*. These clients also maintained muscle mass and lost more body fat than those who didn't eat enough protein.

The function of protein in the body

The body uses proteins for the structure of all body cells, for regulation of many body processes and as a potential source of energy.

The protein structure of each tissue in the body is unique. Each body protein is constructed to perform specific functions and cannot be replaced by other proteins. Adequate protein levels are necessary for building new muscle tissue. Additionally, consuming protein with each meal gives satiety (feeling satisfied).

Proteins consist of chains of amino acids, which are linked to each other. Your body can make some of these amino acids (nonessential amino acids), but there are others that you must eat in your diet (essential amino acids). Essential amino acids are needed to build new proteins which carry out the important functions of your body, such as new muscle, tissue repair, hormone and fluid balance, to name a few.

How protein affects blood sugar levels

When protein foods are eaten, there is very little rise in blood sugar levels, which in turn will cause very little rise in insulin levels. This is a good thing. Because the lower the insulin levels, *the less chance your body will want to store fat.*

Complete and incomplete proteins

Protein sources, which contain all of the essential amino acids, are called "complete proteins." Complete proteins are eggs, milk, cheese, meat, poultry and fish.

Protein sources that lack one or more essential amino acid are called "incomplete." Incomplete proteins are plant foods such as cereals, beans, legumes, nuts and vegetables. Incomplete proteins can be mixed and combined to make a "complete" protein. For example, the main source of protein for vegetarians is plant based, so using a combination of incomplete proteins fill the requirement. With vegetarians, it's difficult to achieve a perfect balance of carbohydrates to protein, mainly because the protein sources also contribute a high amount of carbohydrates. However, egg whites and fish are excellent non-carbohydrate sources of lean proteins.

Recommendations

The recommended DRI's are 10-35 percent of total calories from protein. The "3 Apple-a-Day" Plan recommends 40 percent calories from protein, or one gram per pound body weight (see Nutrient Chart in Chapter 11).

> ***Tip:*** *Include a small amount of a complete protein each time you eat.*

Chapter 9
Fats—Healthy vs. Unhealthy

Good for you? Or not?

Fat is associated with overweight. Billions of dollars are spent annually by people trying to lose those excess layers of body fat. Yet controversy remains on the role fats play in causing disease. Many believe lowering your fat intake will improve health. Others believe replacing "bad" fats with "good" fats will improve health.

Unfortunately, if you are overfat, it is likely that the amount of fat you burn is small, relative to the amount of fat you store. Consequently, the more fat you eat, the more fat you'll store, but this can be changed through diet and exercise.

Saturated fat vs. unsaturated fat

In the study for my Master's Degree thesis, I compared saturated fats versus unsaturated fats and the effect on blood lipids (cholesterol and triglyceride levels) on guinea pigs.

There were four diets, two for each type of fat—saturated and unsaturated. Each was based on a higher level (29 percent of total calories) and lower level (19 percent of total calories) of their respective fats.

The guinea pigs on the higher fat levels from both groups (saturated and unsaturated) had significantly higher visual internal body fat, especially around the organs (heart, liver, kidneys) than the lower fat levels from both groups.

The saturated fat groups also had increased total blood cholesterol compared with the unsaturated fats, which is similar to results of other studies with blood lipid response to the various fats. The triglyceride levels were not significantly different. Although humans are not guinea pigs, we do have similar lipoprotein fractions and metabolism of fats.

Your body's fat requirements

Only a small amount of fat is needed for normal body function and a lower fat diet may aid in maximizing body fat loss. According to Dr. Jequier, writing in the European Journal of Clinical Nutrition, fat intake should not be below *10 percent of the total energy intake* for normal body functions.

How fat functions

Fat is a constituent of the body. The following are some of the functions:

1. Dietary fats provide nine calories per gram of fat. The body's deposits of

fat are a built-in reserve for energy and we have an unlimited amount.

2. Fat is protein-sparing because its availability reduces the need to burn protein for energy.
3. By providing insulation, fats help maintain constant body temperatures.
4. Fats provide cushion for the organs.
5. Fats facilitate the absorption of fat-soluble vitamins A, D, E, and K.

Three classifications of fat

Types of fat include saturated, polyunsaturated and monounsaturated. Saturated fats have been associated with increased risk of heart disease. Saturated fats mostly come from animal sources such as fatty meats and full fat dairy. Polyunsaturated and monounsaturated fats, which usually come from plant sources, have been associated with the reversal of heart disease.

However, some plant oils have been partially hydrogenated (such as margarine) to form trans fatty acids or "bad" fats. Trans fatty acids increase the risk of heart disease by boosting levels of LDL (see Cholesterol in this section). Trans fatty acids are not essential and provide no health benefits.

Why essential fats are…essential!

Essential fats must be present in the diet because the body cannot make them. Two essential fatty acids are linoleic and linolenic.

Linoleic acid, (Omega-6 fatty acids), found in cottonseed oil, safflower oil and sunflower oil, is required for normal growth, healthy skin, transport and metabolism of cholesterol and other bodily functions. The omega-6's are all used heavily in processed foods like crackers, cookies, chips and pastries. Although vital to cellular health, too many omega-6 fatty acids can negate the benefits of omega-3's.

Linolenic acid (Omega-3 fatty acids) is found in salmon, tuna, ground flaxseeds and flaxseed oils. According to Artemis Simopoulos, M.D., director of the Center for Genetics, Nutrition and Health, omega-3's have been found to counter a variety of illnesses and diseases. It is believed that the problem with our modern diet is that it contains far more omega-6 fatty acids than omega-3's causing an imbalance, which makes us more vulnerable to many diseases.

Fat recommendation

The recommended DRI's for total fat is 20-35 percent of the total calories. The "3 Apple-a-Day" Plan is 20 percent of the total calories (see Nutrient Chart in Chapter 11).

The DRI's for essential fats per day are: Omega-6's (linoleic) 12 grams for women and 17 grams for men; Omega-3's (linolenic) 1.1 grams for women and 1.6 grams for men.

Tip: *Fats are high in calories, very concentrated and we need very little. Try to consume fats in their original form (i.e. flaxseeds versus flaxseed oil) or eat three ounces of salmon three times per week or add ground flaxseeds to cereal or protein shakes, as a general rule of thumb. On labels, try to keep no more than two grams of fat per 100 calories.*

Chapter 10
Cholesterol and Triglycerides

What is cholesterol?

Cholesterol is a waxy substance that is often confused with fat. Although cholesterol can be found in high fat foods, its main source is from animals.

Cholesterol is a necessary and important substance in the body. It is a major structural component of all cells in our body and is especially abundant in the nerve and brain cells. It becomes a problem only when it accumulates in the blood. Blood levels—termed blood lipid profile—includes total cholesterol, LDL (Low Density Lipoprotein), HDL (High Density Lipoprotein), and triglycerides.

Total cholesterol is a sum of all blood cholesterol. Total cholesterol is then further broken down to HDL and LDL

LDL's deliver cholesterol to the cells. They are termed "bad" cholesterol because research shows that at high blood levels, they are associated with increasing heart disease.

On the contrary, HDL's pick up cholesterol from arterial plaque reducing their accumulation. HDL's are termed "good" cholesterol because they appear to have a protective influence against heart disease.

Triglycerides, the technical name for fats and oils, are found in our food and our bodies. Triglycerides have many functions such as transporting fat-soluble vitamins and providing an energy source (see Fats in this chapter). However, high levels of triglycerides found in the blood are associated with diabetes and increased risk of heart disease. The following are normal ranges for blood cholesterol and triglyceride levels:

> Total cholesterol < 200 mg/dl
> LDL < 130 mg/dl
> HDL >35 mg/dl
> Triglycerides <200

What affects cholesterol and triglycerides?

Research has shown that eating high cholesterol foods do not increase cholesterol levels in most people. In fact, less than one percent of heart disease patients are actually affected by dietary cholesterol. But they are affected by saturated fats, which many high cholesterol foods are loaded with. So, take a closer look at food labels that say "no cholesterol," because it doesn't mean the food is low in fat. As a matter of fact, many of those items are actually the opposite—high in either saturated or trans fats.

Research has also shown that in total cholesterol, the LDL's are the most influenced by saturated fats and trans fats—causing a significant increase. Common food sources of saturated/trans fats are full-fat animal products, cookies, crackers, bakery goods, snack items and other convenience type foods.

The idea is to lower the LDL's and increase the HDL's. This can be done easily by exercising, and losing excess body fat. Some research indicates that HDL's are also increased by small amounts of alcohol. But, before you run out and buy a six-pack, previous studies suggest that women may not experience the benefit as once thought.

Alcohol can also increase blood levels of triglycerides, too, along with high glycemic carbohydrates such as sugar, corn syrup and other simple sugars. This is not very helpful if your goal is permanent fat loss.

Apples linked to heart health

A Finnish study of 5,133 men and women, ages 30-69 concluded that a high consumption of flavonoids (a substance found in fruits) from apples was directly associated with the lowest risk for coronary mortality.

Another study from the University of California-Davis confirmed that important phytochemicals (a plant substance) in both apples and apple juice prevented oxidation (stickiness) of LDL cholesterol in the arteries. This stickiness causes build-up (plaque), which is harmful and can lead to heart attacks and/or strokes.

So, eat apples for fat loss and better health—your heart will thank you for it!

Chapter 11
Energy, Water and Alcohol

What are your body's energy requirements?

The total energy requirement of the body includes the basal metabolism (rate of expenditure of energy by the body at rest), the amount of voluntary activity, influence of food, the environmental temperature and the special needs for tissue building. I will refer to energy requirements as calories or caloric needs.

How many calories do you really need?

The amount of calories you need varies and is influenced by many things specific to you. Such as your body size, gender, age, lean and body fat composition, body temperature, thyroid function and growth needs. So you can see why one diet does not fit all—even though some of the books would have you think so!

There are several equations you can use to estimate caloric needs, depending on your goals. One, the Harris Benedict equation uses height, weight and age to determine basal energy expenditure and is mainly used in clinical practice. Another estimation equation is based on current body weight times 10 (refer to Nutrient Chart in this chapter).

Energy requirements from equations are only estimations and may need to be adjusted, once again, depending on your goals.

"I owe the success of sticking with this sound nutrition plan to apples. They are the foundation of my food program. I'm a teacher, and after having an apple for a morning snack at school, I noticed there were more and more students bringing apples for their morning snacks too. I now play a game with many of the newly hooked eaters, where I try to guess what type of apple they brought with them for a snack. I can't believe the healthy trend I've started."

Nicole Szeghalmi, age 27, lost 33 lbs.
and over 20 inches.

The "3 Apple-a-Day" Plan
NUTRIENT CHART
for fat loss

Weight pounds	Calories	Protein grams	Carbohydrate grams	Fat grams	Fiber grams	Water 10 oz. glasses
110	1200	110	110	25	25-35	7
120	1200	120	120	27	25-35	8
130	1300	130	130	29	25-35	8
140	1400	140	140	31	25-35	9
150	1500	150	150	33	25-35	9
160	1600	160	160	35	25-35	10
170	1700	170	170	37	25-35	10
180	1800	180	180	40	25-35	11
190	1900	190	190	42	25-35	11
200	2000	200	200	44	25-35	12
220	2200	220	220	48	25-35	13
240	2400	240	240	53	25-35	14
260	2600	260	260	58	25-35	15
280	2800	280	280	62	25-35	16
300	3000	300	300	67	25-35	17

These estimations, however, may be too low or too high. As you become more active and develop your muscle tissue, you may require more calories. Also, once you have reached your fat loss goal, you'll need to increase your calories to maintain it.

How low can your calories go?

Many people believe that to lose weight, you need to lower your calories. This is only partially true. If you keep your calories at your basal energy needs (the minimal amount of calories your body needs to maintain normal function), the increased activity and exercise will create the deficit for fat loss.

On the other hand, if your calories are too low to start, meaning below your basal energy requirements, you will have difficulty making progress. Your body will begin a survival mode, and *conserve and protect its fat stores!* The key is to feed your muscle and not feed your fat. The foods in the "3 Apple-a-Day" Plan are designed to do this.

Eat when you're hungry

Pay attention to your hunger cues. Eat when you are truly hungry. True hunger is when your stomach is "growling" or "rumbling." Many times we are so busy, we don't pay attention to these cues.

Many people often skip breakfast because they don't "feel" hungry in the morning, but *eating breakfast can boost your metabolism and set your blood sugar levels for the day.* Once you establish eating breakfast regularly, it will be difficult to skip.

Caffeine or stimulants can also interfere (delay) those hunger cues. If you do consume caffeine, do so in moderation, one to two cups of coffee or other caffeinated beverages per day.

Tip: *Start with 10 calories per pound of body weight. If you are too full, or feel like you are "stuffing" yourself, lower your calories by 100 per day. If you feel hungry often, increase your calories by 100 per day.*

Water. You can't live without it!

Water is one of the most important nutrients in your life. You can survive for only a few days without it, although you can live weeks without food. Also, inadequate fluid intakes will slow your body's ability to maximize body fat loss.

What water does for your body

In your blood, water transports glucose, oxygen, and fats to working muscles and carries away metabolic by-products, such as carbon dioxide and lactic acid. In the urine, water eliminates metabolic waste products. The darker the urine, the more concentrated the wastes. Water as sweat dissipates the heat through the skin. In the saliva and gastric secretions, water helps digestion. Water also lubricates the joints and cushions organs and tissues.

How much should you drink?

The general recommendations are 8-10 glasses of water per day. I recommend 0.6 ounces per pound body weight of water or non-caloric, non-caffeinated beverages. Yes, the latter items count in your total water consumption, too (see previous Nutrient Chart).

Example: Female 150 pounds x 0.6 ounces = 90 ounces per day

Can alcohol fit into a fat loss program?

Alcohol delivers seven calories per gram. Alcohol also interferes with normal blood sugar levels and fat metabolism. Frequent drinking results in adverse effects on muscle growth. Alcohol decreases protein synthesis and affects Type II muscle fibers (strength type fibers) more than Type I (endurance type fibers.) Excessive alcohol consumption or binge drinking can result in decreased levels of testosterone and increased levels of cortisol (a muscle-destroying hormone), which has a direct effect on muscle cells and can result in significant muscle wasting.

That said, remember what your goals are. *Do you want to run to reach them—or walk?*

Alcohol recommendation

For a fat loss effect, pass on the alcoholic beverages until you've reached your desired body fat level. Then, an occasional drink may not affect your success.

Your body is similar to your car

Imagine your body is your dream car. The type of fuel you put in will determine how well your car (or body) will run. Will you choose supreme fuel or the cheap stuff? Naturally, you would want your dream car to stay in mint condition and last for years. So you would maintain it well, provide it with water for cooling, oil for lubrication and always fill its tank with the best fuel. Your body is similar. Your muscles are the engine which require the necessary fuel (carbohydrates and protein), water (lots) and oil (sparingly) for cooling, lubrication and a myriad of other vital functions.

Do this maintenance religiously and your body (and your car) will run like a dream for your lifetime!

Chapter 12
Metabolic Cost of Food and Meal Frequency

Eating takes energy!

When food is eaten, energy is required to digest and utilize the nutrients from the food. This is called the metabolic cost, or thermogenic effect, of food. The protein, carbohydrates and fats from food all require energy from your body so that you can use the nutrients to continue normal bodily functions.

When you have adequate intake of these nutrients, your body will run efficiently and will be unlikely to store body fat. On the other hand, if you have excess intakes of protein, carbohydrates and fats, *your body will store the excess as body fat*. To make matters even worse, your body will then hang onto the fat and proceed to burn excess carbohydrates and protein.

> ***Tip:*** *If you seem extra hungry on some days, fill up on some extra protein and water and wait 20 minutes. If this doesn't satisfy, add extra vegetables or fruit.*

Eat more to lose!

Timing is of essence when you are trying to lose body fat. Start the "3 Apple-a-Day" Plan with breakfast and eat every two to three hours. The meals are low in fat so your body will burn the calories quickly.

As your muscle tissue develops, your metabolism will also increase and you may get very hungry between meals. Small, frequent meals are a key to keeping your blood sugar and insulin levels stable and constant to maintain your maximum energy level—and minimize the chance of excess calories in a meal to be stored as fat.

Don't skip meals!

Skipping meals or depriving your body of food for long periods of time (other than sleeping) will cause it to access alternative fuel sources to maintain normal body functions. This means your body will use its reserves: first glycogen (stored carbohydrates), then muscle tissue (protein), and the very last, unfortunately, fat.

If this cycle continues, your body will become very good and efficient at storing fat. It's the feast and famine theory. Over time, you will needlessly lose (shrink) your muscle tissue (which decreases your metabolism) and *store more and more body fat.* There's that vicious cycle again!

Breakfast of champions

There's no doubt breakfast is important. A long-term study from Lester Breslow, UCLA School of Public Health, has been following a sample population of 5,000 adults since 1965—about two-thirds of whom have reported their eating and behavioral habits for a decade.

Young adults who said they ate breakfast every day were only half as likely to be obese eight years later. They were equally unlikely to develop insulin resistance syndrome, a metabolic imbalance that can lead to weight gain, Type II Diabetes and heart attack.

Along with this, David Ludwig from Children's Hospital in Boston speculates that a good breakfast keeps blood sugar under control, and filling up in the morning helps manage hunger later in the day.

Not just *any* breakfast will do

When Ludwig fed 12 obese teenage boys breakfast and lunch under controlled conditions, he discovered that even the choice between instant and old-fashioned style oatmeal made a big difference in overeating.

The more rapidly digested, high-carbohydrate meals, including instant oatmeal with sugar—pumped up insulin in the blood and suppressed other hormones leading to hunger and more eating later in the day.

So, what's the bottom line?

Whole grain or high fiber carbohydrates (fruit or vegetables) combined with a good source of protein—eggs, low-fat dairy, or lean meats as laid out in the "3 Apple-a-Day" Plan provide lasting energy. Count on it!

You've reached your goal. Now what?

Often times, losing weight is not as difficult as keeping the weight off (been there, done that?) So it's critical for you to understand—as you go through your fat loss phase—if you want to keep the fat off, most of these changes you've made are to be continued forever!

Yes, forever. *This is the secret to permanent fat loss.*

Why do people gain back their weight?

There are several reasons for this perplexing problem. One of the most common is that they lost weight too fast and a significant part of that weight was muscle. That's why you may want to focus on losing only one to two pounds per week.

Remember, one pound of fat equals 3500 calories that need to be burned. That is a lot of energy to exert for just one pound of fat. If you are losing faster than that, it's likely to be muscle tissue.

Another reason some people gain weight back is they stop exercising once their goal is attained. You must realize that you can't just stop exercising, and/or eating well, and expect your body to maintain.

Finding the balance, as well as how much you can "get away with," (and not gain the weight back) can be tricky.

Tips from clients who have been successful in maintaining their weight loss.
- *Plan a splurge day (maybe a holiday) or one splurge meal (maybe once a week) where you allow yourself to indulge in anything you want.*
- *Continue keeping your food journal no matter how off track you are— you will find a "u-turn" in the process.*
- *Keep exercising but scale back the workout some and take one day a week to rest.*
- *Continue to follow your same meal plans with more variations.*
- *Always keep your water intake on track.*

Life goes on

So what if you lost your focus today? Get back on track with the next meal! Sometimes you have to live a little! You will always have opportunities, such as birthdays, dinner parties, and holidays, to eat foods other than what is listed in the plan.

The key is, to keep in mind what you are striving for and prepare ahead of time for company, parties, holidays and other food-related engagements so that you continue to progress mentally and physically. You can't stop living just because you want to shape up! It's how you prepare and handle those times that will keep you on track.

A lifetime commitment

View this new plan as your journey or challenging adventure that will get easier as time passes, if you stay focused. I really believe holidays (the official ones listed on the calender—not making your own!) are the time to splurge, and the rest of the time you can stay focused on keeping your body strong and healthy!

As a side benefit, those special events will be even more enjoyable, thanks to the self-confidence and pride that your new strong, healthy, good-looking body will bring to your life.

Chapter 13

Dining Out, Portion Control, Convenience and Supplements

Let someone else do the cooking!

Dining out can be an enjoyable experience. So there's no reason to hibernate when you are on a fat loss program. Especially when it can easily fit into your meal plan.

All you have to do is follow the tips below and be firm when you order. Most restaurants are quite used to people on special diets and are happy to accommodate your needs. Remember, you are the one picking up the check—and leaving the tip!

Tips *for dining out:*
* *Always order salad dressing on the side. Ask for low-calorie or fat free dressing.*
* *With pasta, rice, or baked potato, ask for sauce, butter, sour cream or other high fat toppings on the side.*
* *When ordering meat, choose grilled chicken breast or fish.*
* *Avoid deep fried or fried foods. They're not only loaded with fat and low in nutrients, they usually contain trans fats or "bad" fats.*
* *Ask for stir-fry without oil.*
* *Instead of the regular sides, ask for double steamed vegetables.*
* *Mexican food—request whole beans instead of refried. Ask for cheese, sour cream and guacamole on the side. Order chicken fajitas and use corn tortillas instead of flour.*
* *Fast food choices—order a grilled chicken breast sandwich with no sauces, or salads without cheese and low-cal salad dressing.*
* *Order pizza without cheese or cut the amount of cheese in half. Choose vegetable toppings or lean Canadian bacon. Order extra thin crust.*

"Super-size" portions. More than you bargained for?

Our society whole-heartedly embraces the notion that bigger is better. You can "super size" almost any fast food item inexpensively—it's called "value-marketing." It seems to make economical sense, too, as you get more food for very little extra cost. The real expense may come later if you have to deal with medical bills from overfat-related diseases. Unfortunately, they don't "super-size" health care costs these days.

A study conducted by health organizations nationwide, including the American Institute for Cancer Research, attempted to quantify how much damage "value marketing" does. Here are some of their findings:

- At McDonald's, researchers paid eight cents *less* to buy the large value meal (Quarter Pounder with cheese, large fries and large Coke at 1,380 calories) than a Quarter Pounder, small fries and small Coke (890 calories). In other words, eight cents *less* to purchase 490 *more* calories.
- When study participants ordered a medium popcorn without butter (900 calories) in a movie theater, they were "upsold" to a large popcorn (1,160 calories) for only 60 cents more—23 percent *more* money for 260 *more* calories.
- At 7-Eleven, researchers asking for a "Gulp" of Coke (150 calories) left the store with a "Double Gulp" (600 calories) for only 37 cents more— a 42 percent increase in price for *400 percent more calories.*
- At another fast food restaurant, a study participant asked for a cheese-burger and was "upsold" to a meal package—cheeseburger, fries and a Coke—for only $1.40 more. Even "better" she could "super-size" that meal for only 58 cents more. Her lunch now contained 1,380 calories, or about 700 *more* calories than a woman her size requires at lunch.

Are you portion challenged?

Food and beverage portions have grown over the past few years in restaurants, grocery items and even at home. Many people do not have a clue as to what a normal portion size should be.

So when you begin this Plan, take the time to measure your food accurately—it's very important to get a realistic picture of what you're actually consuming. Use food scales, measuring cups and measuring spoons. You'll soon begin to identify portion sizes just by looking. In fact, most people get the hang of it within a few weeks—and so will you!

Here are some other visual techniques for gauging portions if you are dining out:

1 serving of vegetables or fruit = a closed fist
1 ounce of cheese = two extended fingers
1 cup of dry cereal = a cupped hand
1 serving (three ounces) of meat = size of the palm of your hand
1 teaspoon of butter = tip of your thumb

> **Tip:** *Measure your foods accurately throughout this Plan. Your efforts will create worthwhile results.*

Weight loss is not always "convenient"

We are a fast food nation and our society seems to want more and more convenience. We have the technology to provide it too, but this same convenience is one of the major contributing factors in making us fatter.

Achieving *permanent fat loss* sometimes is not convenient. Although the apples in this plan do provide convenience, learning to cook and prepare meals ahead of time will add even more convenience, not to mention taste better—and you'll know what's in it!

> **Tip:** *Use your grocery store, not the drive thru window, to buy wholesome foods.*

Potato chips and couch potatoes

I wrote a letter to the President last year asking for a nationwide, federally funded, "get-in-shape" contest. The purpose was to help combat our escalating obesity problem by motivating people to get off their couches, put on their gym shorts—and eat more fruits and vegetables.

Do you know that the majority of marketing dollars are spent on junk food (which makes us fatter) and the least amount is spent on produce (fruits and vegetables)? Yet we scratch our heads and wonder why Americans are getting fatter—not to mention more sedentary. Hello?

More fat people are on the way, too. You'll see why if you ever watch TV programming for kids, which features one junk food commercial after another (with no fruit and vegetable commercials at all!)

Although I did not get a reply from Washington, anyone can write and encourage suggestions for national health improvements. If enough people speak up, someone will hear.

Do you need supplements to succeed in this plan?

Not on the "3 Apple-a-Day" Plan. As a dietitian, I believe food is the best source of fuel for optimizing fat loss. Food is what helps our bodies recreate. However, with the lower calorie levels (1200, 1500), I do recommend a multivitamin/mineral supplement and additional calcium for most people even if their diet is the best it can be.

A vitamin/mineral/calcium supplement is not a replacement for a poor diet, but an enhancement to a very good diet. In this Plan, I suggest a shake that requires protein powder as a snack. This suggestion is primarily for convenience and not a necessity. The protein shake can easily be substituted with another meal option. Protein powders can be from whey, egg whites or soy.

As for other sports enhancement supplements, I do not recommend them in your efforts to maximize fat loss. Many of the fat loss products or thermogenics on the market are not regulated by the FDA and may be unsafe. I recommend *apples as your fat loss supplement* to keep your hunger under control.

Moderate caffeine (one to two cups of brewed coffee per day, or 300 mg of caffeine) can enhance both performance and endurance. Caffeine releases free fatty acids, which can provide additional energy for the workout. On the other hand, too much caffeine can interfere with calcium and other nutrient absorption. Too much caffeine can also delay the hunger response (or cue to eat), which may cause you to overeat later.

Tip: *Eating equal amounts of protein and carbohydrate plus exercise will give you the greatest fat loss results.*

Key Points for Part III

- Make the foundation of each meal a fruit and/or vegetable, lean protein and water.
- Consume one gram each of lean protein and low-glycemic carbohydrate per pound body weight per day.
- Fiber should be at least 25-35 grams per day. Three apples provide 15 grams alone.
- Eat three ounces of salmon, three times per week, for your essential fats.
- Start with 10 calories per pound current weight for calorie needs.
- Drink at least 8-10 ounce glasses of water per day.
- Eat breakfast and four to five small meals every day to keep metabolism and energy level optimum.
- Measure your food in the beginning for accurate portions.
- Use apples as your fat loss supplement, one before each major meal.

PART IV

Exercise—a Key to Staying Young

❖

Physical Activity vs. Exercise

Exercise and Permanent Fat Loss

❖

Chapter 14
Physical Activity vs. Exercise

So there's a difference?

Actually, yes. Recently, there have been several recommendations for the amount and types of exercise or physical activity needed to be healthy and/or to experience weight loss. Specialists have long advised 30 minutes of moderately intense physical activity every day for overall health. Recently, the Institute of Medicine's (DRI's) new exercise goal is one hour per day, seven days per week. This recommendation is based on how much energy is expended from an individual of a healthy weight.

Physical activity includes walking the dog, house cleaning, stair climbing, playing catch with the kids and other moving activities. Exercise is an exertion of mind and body for development and training. Exercise is being consciously active with a purpose.

Many (especially women) believe that weight lifting will give them big, bulky muscles. Although there are some that will develop obvious muscle faster, it's not likely that you will get big and bulky. The key is activating the muscle tissue and losing the fat layer on top of the muscle so you will have a leaner, sleeker body.

Chapter 15

Exercise and Permanent Fat Loss

Exercise is work! When can I lighten up?

Let's clear the air on the whole exercise issue. It's not a temporary activity you do when you are on a "diet." To achieve permanent fat loss, you need to activate and build your lean muscle tissue—and maintain it throughout your life. There's just no getting around it!

My grandmother, 90 years young, lives alone and exercises at the gym three times per week and can out walk any 50-year-old in town. Not only that, she's in better health, both mentally and physically, than many 50-year-olds! By the way, she eats at least one apple per day and includes fruits and vegetables with every meal.

Increasing your muscle tissue increases your metabolism, or metabolic rate (your ability to burn calories). The more you increase your muscle tissue and therefore metabolism, the more calories you'll burn—even while you are sleeping!

Your body was designed to be active. Today's environment has made it too easy to be sedentary—long commutes, elevators, computer-dominated jobs, remote controls, video games, the list goes on and on. According to the Centers for Disease Control and Prevention, nearly four out of 10 adults report getting no exercise at all! Despite the legitimate worry over super-sized portions and junk food, some scientists argue that the nation's obesity epidemic is mostly due to inactivity.

So let's get moving!

Two types of exercise

Basically, there are two major types of exercise your body needs for permanent fat loss results: weight training and cardiovascular training. Stretching, functional training (moving in all ranges of motion with weights) and other types of training (martial arts, yoga etc.) are also important additions for cross training. All activity is good!

Weight training

Weight training, or resistance exercise, is used to strengthen the muscle and maintain or increase muscle tissue. One of the biggest benefits of weight training is that you "wake-up" muscle cells that would not otherwise activate with any other exercise. This creates more metabolically active tissue and increases your body's ability to burn calories. Weight training also strengthens the muscles around your bones, making you less prone to injury.

Research at the University of Alabama shows that just three strength-training sessions per week can help you burn 150 more calories every day—enough to shed 16 pounds of body fat a year.

Keeping your muscle tissue as you age is the key to staying active so you don't become disabled! After the age of 25, we can lose about one percent of muscle mass per year (see example in Chapter 3). According to Tufts University scientists, muscle loss is more universal than osteoporosis. As you lose muscle, you lose strength. When you lose strength, you lose the ability to be active and energetic. With weight training, you can increase your muscle mass at any age.

In other words, "use it or lose it."

Cardiovascular training

Cardiovascular training strengthens the heart and improves the efficiency of the cardiovascular and respiratory system. Certain cardiovascular exercises, termed "weight-bearing" (bearing your own body weight)—brisk walking, running, dancing, stair-climbing and playing sports with your kids—can all help keep you fit and promote bone mass. Best of all, if you are on a mission to lose weight, cardiovascular training is very effective in helping you lose that stubborn, unhealthy extra fat layer.

Train according to your fitness level

Weight training and cardiovascular training should both be gauged according to fitness level. If you're a beginner, you'll need to condition your muscles, joints, and tendons gradually. If you've weight trained in the past but haven't been active for a while, you can ease into it over a few weeks. If you've been consistent with an exercise program, you may be ready to take it to the next level.

> *Always check with your physician before starting an exercise program, especially if you have had previous health risks.*

Exercise recommendations

Beginner: weight train three times per week starting with lighter weights and higher repetitions. Cardiovascular training should be performed four to five times per week for 20 minutes per day. As you become more fit, you'll need to increase your intensity (effort) and weights (see Beginner Exercise Program in the Appendix).

Intermediate: weight train three to four times per week. You'll want a program that is progressive and has a variety of exercises, repetitions and sets.

Cardiovascular training should be five times per week for 30-40 minutes per day.

Advanced: weight train four times per week with heavier weights, less repetitions. Perform cardiovascular training five to six days per week for 30-45 minutes per day.

The "3 Apple-a-Day" Plan

Exercise Guidelines for Fat Loss

	Weight Training Sessions per week	Cardiovascular Training Sessions per week/time	Stretching Sessions per week
Beginner	3	4-5 sessions/20 minutes	5
Intermediate	4	5 sessions/30-40 minutes	5
Advanced	4	5-6 sessions/30-45 minutes	daily

Tip: *Think of exercise as your prescription for survival. If you don't exercise, you'll shorten your active life. All activity of movement, from house cleaning to weight training, is accumulative and will improve your health.*

Key Points for Part IV

- Exercise is essential for permanent fat loss.
- Weight training will increase lean muscle tissue. Increased muscle tissue will increase metabolism.
- Cardiovascular training will help you lose the existing excess fat layer.
- All physical activity can improve your health. Inactivity contributes to being overfat.

PART V

Success Stories

❖

Personal Success Stories

Quick Start

Phases

FAQ's

❖

Nicole Szeghalmi, age 27

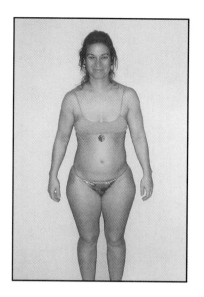 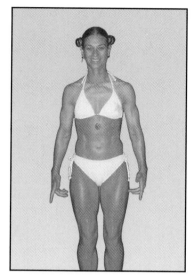

	Before	After	Change
Weight/pounds	140	107	-33
Body fat percent	26	11	-15
Waist	32”	24”	-8”
Hips	40”	33”	-7”
Thigh	24”	19”	-5”

I owe the success of sticking with a sound nutrition plan ("3 Apple-a-Day" Plan) to apples. They were the foundation of my food program. There isn't any type of apples I haven't tried. As long as they're fresh, I'm happy.

The toughest time for me to stick to my healthy eating program was during the evening. I just love to snack at night. So I used apples to satisfy my snack cravings. The apples quieted the rumblings in my belly without weighing me down with a bunch of calories.

Every aspect of my life has improved. The twelve-week challenge has had such a positive impact on the way I live my life that the list may cause me to run out of paper. Here is a list of my top seven that I consider to be the most improved:

1. Knee pain: I have had two surgeries and living daily with knee pain until now. I think the combination of losing weight and building strength gave my knee better support, relieving the pain.
2. Ability to self-motivate: I now believe that with hard work and dedication, I can accomplish any goals I set for myself.
3. Skin complexion: because of my food program, my complexion has

cleared up and it looks healthy.

4. Increased energy: I have a lot of energy throughout the day now, whereas before I was taking naps.

5. Increased strength: I love how I can qualitatively track my progress with weights. In the beginning, I could barely lift 10-pound dumbbells while performing lunges and now I can handle 30 pounds!

6. Increased feeling of well-being: since I have been working out, my mood has improved giving me a higher ability to cope with stresses, both good and bad. Therefore, I have a more positive outlook on life.

7. Increased self-confidence: my clothes seem to fit better now and I don't feel like running and hiding when I have on my bikini.

So now I come to an end with this awesome experience. Life-changing experience would better describe it and I have nothing but positive words and thoughts about it. I can't believe how fast the 12 weeks have passed. Although it was tough at times, I wouldn't trade it for anything. I look for ward to new challenges.

Nicole won 1st place and $50,000 in the national Gold's Gym Challenge, 2003.

Stacey Lienemann, age 23

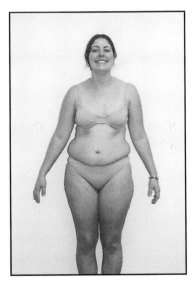 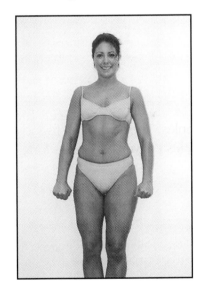

	Before	After	*Change*
Weight/pounds	172	143	-29
Body fat percent	33	21	-12
Waist	35.5"	31.25"	-4.25"
Hips	44.25"	38"	-6.25"
Thigh	26"	23"	-3"

The Gold's Gym Challenge has changed my life dramatically. It's hard to imagine that a short 12 weeks ago I was an unhappy, unhealthy and overweight 23 year-old mother of one, Jaden, my daughter who is 16 months old.

I have always imagined myself as an active happy mother with bounds of energy, strength and creativity. Twelve weeks ago, I found myself at 175 pounds, tired, angry and unhappy with my life. My family was suffering because of the way I was. My dream was to change my activities and eating habits to enable myself to become healthier, both physically and mentally.

I knew that if I didn't do something to change my life soon I may never change it at all. Going through life unhappy and lazy is one of my biggest fears. That fear is what pushed me into the gym. I decided to enter the "Get-in-Shape" contest.

I put myself on a six-day-a-week workout plan that consisted of a variety of different classes. I also incorporated up to an hour of cardio a day.

I expected the beginning days to be grueling. Lack of self-esteem, energy and strength makes everything seem difficult. However, my drive and determination to become healthier and more physically fit motivated me tremendously. I didn't want to be the girl in the back of the class that gets winded after the warm up. So, I stuck with it and before long, I began to gain strength and endurance. When I finished a class, I could feel my self-esteem grow and my butt shrink. The stronger I grow the more I am able to push myself. The classes enabled me to have fun with my workout, and having a set time to be at the gym gave me the discipline I need to continue my progress.

When it comes to dieting, discipline is my major problem. Eating has always been a challenge for me because I eat when I'm bored. If I'm not bored then I'm busy and I will forget to eat all together.

The "3 Apple-a-Day" Plan made me realize what our bodies need to function. Realizing that food is fuel for your body helped me change my eating habits forever. Now instead of eating because I'm bored, I eat to fuel my muscles and produce energy. The more knowledge I gain about food and what it does for our bodies the easier it is to pick healthy food choices.

In the past 12 weeks, I have become addicted to going to the gym first thing every day. My life has changed tremendously because of this contest. I love myself now and that is the best prize I could ever receive. I can feel my dreams starting to come true. I am a fit, motivated, happy 23-year old mother of one and I am extremely proud of myself for accomplishing my goals.

Stacey won 1st place and $2,200 in Gold's Gym of Wenatchee local contest, 2003.

Jason Mathews, age 27

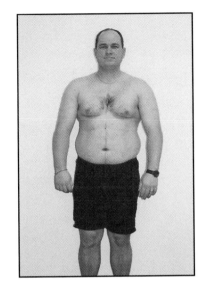 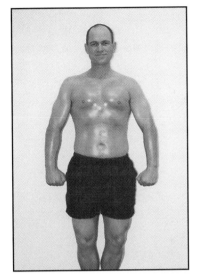

	Before	After	Changes
Weight/pounds	258	199	-59
Body fat percent	42	11	-31
Waist	45.75"	36"	-9.75"
Hips	46.5"	40.5"	-6"
Thigh	29.5"	24"	-5.5"

I had two big motivators to join the contest, my dad and my wife. About two years ago, my dad was diagnosed with diabetes and a large cancerous tumor in one of his kidneys. He had to make an immediate lifestyle change—eating healthier, exercising and losing weight. He has been successful and is cancer free.

My wife was diagnosed with Leukemia over three years ago. At 25, this was a total shock to both of us. The treatment damaged her hip and required a hip replacement. Through her entire ordeal, we both gained a lot of weight.

I used to be involved in sports and other activities and believed I was still in okay shape. Then I had a body composition test that revealed just how out of shape I had become. I was determined to get back into shape. My wife and I began our quest to become fit together.

What I really enjoyed was the immediate results from the diet and exercise program provided to us by Gold's Gym. I lost 12 pounds the first week. I always thought food had to have grease and fat to taste good, until we began cooking some of the recipes, especially the chili, provided by Tammi Flynn. My wife and I both learned how to use fresh fruits and vegetables in our diet. We now plan and prepare foods to take with us to work.

During the contest, my wife and I learned a lot about will power. If one of us thought about cheating, the other quickly steered that person back into the right direction.

The best thing now is to hear people ask my wife and I how much weight we have lost. And telling us that we look great!

Jason lost 85 pounds of fat and gained 26 pounds of muscle! He won 1st place and $2,200 in Gold's Gym of Wenatchee's local contest, 2003.

❖ ❖ ❖

Vicki Robins, age 32

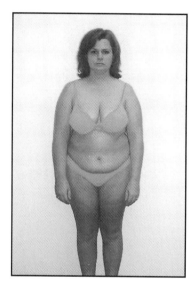 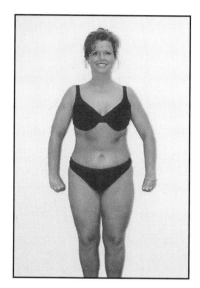

	Before	After	Changes
Weight/pounds	158	134	-24
Body fat percent	39	30.5	-8.5
Waist	40.25"	32.5"	-7.75"
Hips	41.5"	38"	-3.5"
Thigh	26"	23.25"	-2.75"

"Mommy, if having babies in your tummy make it big like yours, I don't want to have any," said my six-year old daughter. I knew then that I needed to do something to change my eating habits. It is one thing to accept the image of a frumpy mom of three, but to hear these words is a "big" eye opener and very painful. I never knew my being overweight affected my children this way. I am a "stay-at-home" mom and give my children all of me, but did not realize, in a sense, that was too much. I want to be a positive role model in every way to my children and the weight I was at was not only harming me, but them as well.

When I looked at my "before" pictures, I was amazed and disgusted at how

I had let myself go. The front pose is something I looked at every day and had become used to, but the back pose shocked me! This was the biggest motivator I needed. The times I felt like giving up, I just looked at my pictures, and that kept me going.

The words *"discipline versus willpower"* were constant in my thoughts. Also the pictures from past contestants gave me a boost when I needed one. To know that moms just like me had greatly improved their figures, I knew I could do the same.

When I began eating healthier, everyone in my family benefited. I went from buying 21 apples per week to double that amount. My oldest daughter began reading labels and made sure I did not eat anything that was unacceptable in my new way of eating.

We, as a family, are also more active. All five of us are starting softball and loving the exercise together.

In 12 weeks, I attained all of my goals and then some. My daughter now realizes it is a choice to be frumpy and not a result of pregnancy. I find I am a better wife and mother for it and hope that my children will understand the importance of fitness. I can't wait to see what the next 12 weeks will bring. If I can do it, anyone can!

Vicki won 1st place and $2,200 in Gold's Gym of Wenatchee's local contest, 2003.

Tim Kiele, age 35

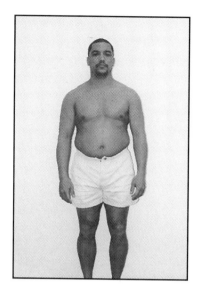 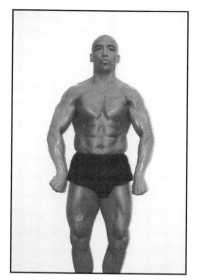

	Before	After	Changes
Weight/pounds	178	155	-22
Body fat percent	15	7	-8
Waist	37.25"	31.5"	-5.75"
Hips	41"	36"	-5"
Thigh	24.75"	23"	-1.75"

There are two reasons why I chose to take the challenge at Gold's Gym. A neck injury, accompanied by bulging discs in my lower back—which have hindered my life. And the neds of my family.

Twelve years ago, wheen I met my wife, I played national flag football, basketball, softball and golfed. My dream was to become a daddy, and I was blessed with twin daughters. Never did I think I would have to utter the words, "Sorry babies, daddy's back hurts and he can't play right now." This had to stop. I owed it to my wife and children to turn my life around.

During the contest, I noticed dramatic changes in my body, which I attribute to the "3 Apple-a-Day" Plan. Implementing apples alone was a step in the right direction. Eating apples caused me to eat less and have been great substitutes between meals. I will continue to eat them on a daily basis!

I had a lot of support throughout the contest. Working graveyard has made it impossible to get a "good nights sleep." So one could imagine the challenge on some days—just making it to the gym, let alone getting in a good workout. The smiles and support of the staff created such positive energy that it gave me the boost I needed to push even harder towards the goals I had set for myself.

Those 12 weeks, through the contest, have given me back that "fire" I had prior to my injuries. Now that I have reached all my personal goals, I intend to set future goals, which include helping my family live a healthier and happier lifestyle with me.

Tim won 1st place and $2,200 in Gold's Gym of Wenatchee's local contest and 3rd place in the national Gold's Gym Challenge, 2003.

❖   ❖   ❖

Maureen Ropp, age 48

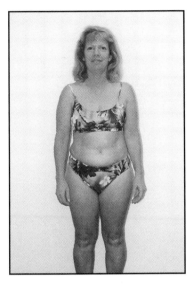 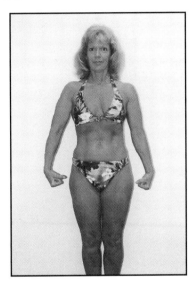

	Before	After	Changes
Weight/pounds	143	120	-23
Body fat percent	32	23	-9
Waist	32.75"	29.25"	-3.5"
Hips	41"	36"	-5"
Thigh	24.5"	22"	-2.5"

I started this contest with my husband because we wanted to be healthier, and we could see ourselves gradually going in the wrong direction. We didn't want our physical health to limit what we could do—we wanted to choose our own lifestyles, our health, our own future and quality of life!

We found that *planning and preparation* is the key to success. We kept journals or our training, plus we used a program to track our calorie intake. We found you must measure and weigh everything until you learn proper portion sizes. We ate five to six meals per day and ate our three apples every day (my favorite is Fuji). We kept our fat intake to less than 20 percent of total calories, and balanced our remaining calories between carbohydrates and protein (as in the "3 Apple-a-Day" Plan). I have been very fortunate to have a very supportive husband who has helped me with training and food preparation. It's also great to have support from your family and friends.

We have set a personal goal of riding the 200 mile STP, Seattle to Portland, bike ride in July. I never imagined two years ago that I would be able to accomplish even a 20-mile ride. I was winded just climbing the stairs and my joints were starting to swell with soreness. Now I'm climbing hills with my bike!

If you learn how good you can feel and how much you can accomplish, regardless of age, then you definitely are a winner! I know I am!

Maureen won 1st place and $2,200 in Gold's Gym of Wenatchee's local contest, 2003.

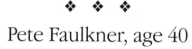

Pete Faulkner, age 40

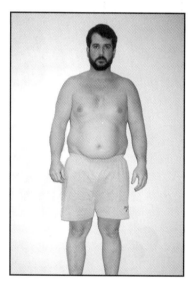 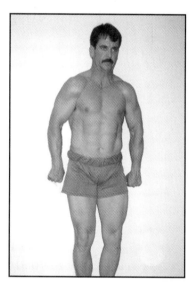

	Before	After	Changes
Weight/pounds	215	173	-42
Body fat percent	28	9	-19
Waist	45"	34"	-11"
Hips	45.5"	38"	-7.5"
Thigh	29"	23.5"	-5.5"

I am a bricklayer by trade, as my father was and his father as well. I was raised amongst men, what you would call a "man's man." I've been married for 16 years to a beautiful wife who gave me two children and stuck with me through thick and thin. I felt my wife needed more of a husband and father than what I had become.

I was 50 pounds overweight. It hurt to get up in the morning. I could barely lay brick all day. After work, all I could do was lay on the couch and watch TV. My children needed me to communicate and be active, but it just wasn't there. I would toss and turn all night. Some mornings I was more tired when I got up than when I had gone to bed. I was constantly ornery. I ate aspirin like it was candy because my back and hips hurt constantly. I had no emotions about me and I knew, at this rate, I would be burned out soon.

The new year rolled around and I decided to go to Gold's Gym to see what it was all about. I met with a trainer and told him I had never been in a gym before. I also told him I had never been athletic and he assured me not to worry. He said it would be fun. At the time, I did not see any fun in lifting weights and getting on the treadmill, but I signed up anyway.

The first week was tough on me. I was running on the treadmill in $10 K-mart shoes and they raised blisters the size of golf balls on my feet. I knew there would be other obstacles to overcome and the blisters were just one of them.

The second week I started the "3 Apple-a-Day" Plan. I always hated the word "diet" because I had been on so many. But eating real food, six times a day, plus one gallon of water felt good. This was a good plan for me. However, it was challenging when my wife and kids ordered pizza that first Friday. But I wasn't going to sacrifice the three pounds I had lost that week to pizza, so I settled for turkey and rice.

The fourth week the alarm went off at 5 a.m. I sat up and noticed this morning was different. I felt good. I slept through the night and felt laughter and happiness. I wanted to go to the gym…I needed my exercise now!

The day came that I will never forget. The guys in the locker room noticed I'd lost a lot of weight and encouraged me to keep it up. That made me feel good. My energy level was in overdrive and the harder I worked, the better I felt. The better I felt, the harder I worked. From that day on, my feeling towards myself and people had changed. I had a love for the gym and the people around me.

Now, I get up at 5 a.m., prepare my food for the day, go to the gym then to work—and enjoy it! I come home from work, cook dinner, take my son to baseball, return home and do homework with the kids. I then finish my work, visit with my family and head to bed at 10 p.m. My energy level is always very positive and high!

I took first place in the Gold's Gym "Get-in-Shape" contest losing 47 pounds and 19 percent body fat!

Pete won 1st place and $5000 in Gold's Gym of Wenatchee's local contest, 2000, and 4th place in the national Gold's Gym Challenge, 2003.

Sandi Anderson, age 54

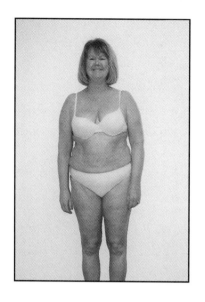 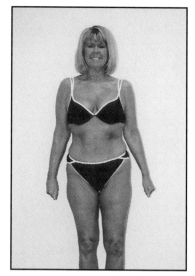

	Before	After	Changes
Weight/pounds	198	169	-29
Body fat percent	41	34	-7
Waist	39.5"	34.75"	-4.75"
Hips	43.25"	40.75"	-2.75"
Thigh	26.75"	24.25"	-2.5"

"You just have a 'slow metabolism'…It's simple, take in less calories, exercise more…you're 'over 50'… you're not expected to be in shape."

These are just a few of the so-called "facts of life" I have listened to my entire life. Having been told by so many that my metabolism is slow, I believed them. Guess what? I now know the truth. I have an above average metabolism, and all these years my body thought it was starving!

As for taking in less calories and exercising more, what a vicious cycle that is. I would start an exercise program and diet, cutting calories to less than half of the required fuel just to function through a normal day. After a few days, I was so exhausted, I would cut out the exercise, so of course I had to cut out some more calories to compensate! I lost weight, but felt awful and ALWAYS gained it back!

After seeing results from past contestants, I thought, if they can do it so can I! To the shock of many people, I decided to go for it. I have learned so much about myself in 12 weeks. The knowledge about how my body works, why I have fought my weight my whole life, and how to maintain a healthy, fit body. This is the knowledge I have been searching for.

The "3 Apple-a-Day" Plan was so easy to follow. I was never hungry. In fact, I had to retrain myself to eat enough. Never tiring of three apples a day, I had no cravings for sweets—I believe the Fuji apples helped in this area. I looked forward to having my apple as a snack every evening! I had more energy, and was amazed at how steadily I lost weight. I plan to continue using the "3 Apple-a-Day" Plan to maintain my weight.

I am so proud of myself! I hope I can motivate another "50- something" to take charge and be the best they can!

Just a small note. Before I started the challenge, I was suffering from "hot flashes" day and night. They have now stopped completely! It's wonderful to be free from that!

Sandi won 1st place and $2,200 in Gold's Gym or Wenatchee's local contest, 2003.

❖   ❖   ❖

Donald Housden, age 55

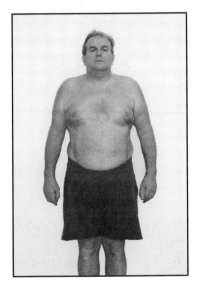 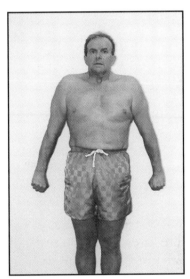

	Before	After	Changes
Weight/pounds	235	201	-34
Body fat percent	35	26	-9
Waist	48.5"	41.25"	-7.25"
Hips	49.25"	43.5"	-5.75"
Thigh	24"	22.75"	-1.75"

It was easy to rationalize my obese body when I was spammed by hundreds of TV and radio ads daily helping me feed my food addiction. I had been over-weight and out of shape for years and accepted life as it was. I was comfortable and in total denial of my "non-existent" problem. You would think at 250 pounds, shortness of breath and Type II Diabetes, I would have a clue!

My wake up call was when my doctor told me after my blood tests, that he could no longer help me—I had to help myself. What a concept! I was to be accountable for my own fate. The way I was doing it now had to change, or else.

I know practice is how to be good at what you do. So I started practicing being an athlete in training. I started a food journal, joined the gym and went daily, aggressively training at being an athlete. I bought athlete clothes, so I could look like an athlete and I would change into them as soon as I got home from work. I even wore them on my days off so I could feel like an athlete. So what, if I look like the Pillsbury Doughboy, in my mind, I was an athlete.

The third week in the program, I had my blood work done again. My doctor thought the lab had sent the wrong results because of such drastic changes; Cholesterol was 361, now 140; triglycerides were 721, now 117. My risk factor for cholesterol fractions went from 6.2, now 2.6. The best results were from my glucose meter, which started at a high of 445 and now was running in the 90 range—*without medication*! I knew I was on the right track!

I started to train even harder after the test results. I brushed off my bicycle, bought a stopwatch, and started riding like an athlete—setting goals and counting my spins per minute. I now ride my bike to the gym, making a round of 11 miles and I love it!

During my seventh week of training, we had an attempted robbery early at work one morning—a really bad person tried to duct tape our bookkeeper and rob the safe. The bookkeeper screamed and at first I thought she had seen a spider. But when she screamed the second time I leaped from the cash register and ran towards the office. I saw a person dressed in black running from the office. You have two seconds to make a judgment call. I, with the help of another employee, captured the robber and called the police. I felt like the guy on the Gold's Gym mural (a buffed athlete). I realized I was no longer an athlete in training, but that I had become an athlete.

I have just begun. I have set new goals and have new challenges to meet. I have my youth back and my life has been restored. I will continue on this journey.

Donald won "Most Inspirational" Award and a new mountain bike in Gold's Gym of Wenatchee's local contest, 2003.

West Mathison, age 26

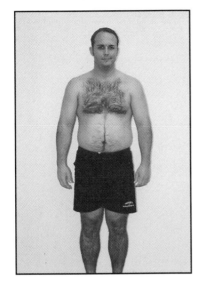 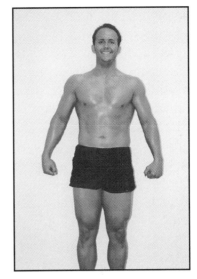

	Before	After	Changes
Weight/pounds	217	185	-32
Body fat percent	22	11	-11
Waist	40.5"	34.25"	-6.25"
Hips	44.25"	39.75"	-4.75"
Thigh	26.25"	24"	-2.25"

Tips on apples and traveling

During the contest, I traveled all but three weeks and was typically gone three days a week. Plus, I wasn't in a position to stop by a grocery store. Therefore, I had a little strategy to keep me consistent. Also, giving myself choices and keeping variety in my diet helped me stay consistent.

Travel days

I'd line the bottom of my briefcase with three apples for my day of travel. During in-flight meals or at customer dinners, I'd pull an apple out of my briefcase just before eating or as we'd walk into the restaurant. My variety selection was based on the characteristics. The Cameo, Granny, Red Delicious or Pink Lady traveled best because they hold a better crunch at room temperature.

Non-travel days

While I was away from home, I would pack (cold) refrigerated apples in my briefcase to be eaten once I arrived at my office. I would pack either Golden Delicious or Galas to refrigerate at my office. These type of apples have a thin skin and are more sensitive to warm temperatures and bruising. They too can travel, but they need protection. While they were still cold, I would put them in a sock (clean sock!) and pack them in my suitcase. They usually keep cool until the end of the day.

Tips to add variety

If I was at home or office, I'd slice an apple and use spices like chili powder, cinnamon and/or allspice to further the variety to my diet.

For me, having variety and creativity kept me consistent with my food plan. I did not get bored with eating apples. With all the new varieties available, I had one for any mood. Having choices made the plan seem unlimited and unregimented.

West won 2nd place and $1,525 in Gold's Gym of Wenatchee's local contest, 2003.

Quick Start

You've read the book, you've heard the recommendations and you believe the "3 Apple-a-Day" Plan is right for you. Now, are you ready to get started on *your journey to permanent fat loss?*

If so, congratulations! Here are the steps to get you going.

Step 1: Set your goal(s). Maybe you have one main goal, but also set mini goals to achieve your main goal.

Step 2: Determine your calorie needs. Start with 10 calories per pound of body weight.

Step 3: Decide if you want to use the entire seven-day meal plan or just one or two days. Find your appropriate calorie level.

Step 4: Buy and prepare your food for the week.

Step 5: Take your measurements and/or your pictures.

Step 6: Start your exercise program.

Step 7: Begin journaling.

Step 8: Stay focused and measure your progress every two weeks.

Step 9: Ask for support through family and friends.

Step 10: HAVE FUN!

Feeling overwhelmed?

Try easing into the plan by taking one step at a time through five phases. To start, think about what you'd like to achieve (a goal). Is your goal to improve appearance, health and/or physical fitness?

Phase 1– Week 1

To figure out what changes are needed to improve your behaviors, make a point of writing down what you do throughout your day. Be specific and include as much as you can. You can also narrate it on a small tape recorder.

After you have completed a couple of days, make two columns, one column for food and beverage and the other for activity. Incorporate the events of your previous days in these columns and continue to do so daily from then on.

Phase 2–Week 2-3

Look at your columns and decide what you want to work on the most—food/beverage or activity.

For food improvement, start by simply drinking more water this week. Gradually increase the amount by one cup to reach your suggested amount (see Nutrient Chart in Chapter 11).

For activity, find 10 minutes in your day and start walking (in or out of your house), or playing with your kids, doing chores—simply moving. Dedicate these 10 minutes every day just to becoming more active.

Phase 3–Week 3-8

Food intakes. Look at how many times you eat fruits and vegetables in the day. If none, it may take a while to reach the recommended amount. Again, start small—add one apple each day for one week. By three weeks, you will be up to three apples per day. Include vegetables in the evenings also. Within four to five weeks, you will be up to the nine suggested servings of produce.

Activity. Now is the time to add some weight training. Your recent activity has conditioned your joints, and it's time to work the muscles to help increase your bone density and metabolism. You can do it from home—get an exercise video or a good home training guide (such as—*Body for Life*). You also may consider finding a health club. A good health club can help guide you and ensure that you perform exercises safely.

Phase 4–Week 9-12

Food. Now let's look at your carbohydrate intake. Carbohydrates come from breads, cereals, crackers, pasta, rice, fruits, vegetables and more. Do you consume large quantities of these? Are carbohydrates (excluding fruits and vegetables) the main food you eat—either snacking or eating a meal? (See emotional triggers Part II). If so, you'll want to start including more protein. Protein foods, such as lean meats, poultry, fish, and low-fat dairy (yogurt, milk, cheese) will help keep your blood sugars stable so you won't keep eating more and more carbohydrates. This will take some planning and thought. Look at your columns and determine how many times you are eating protein and how many times you are eating carbohydrates. Try making them equal.

Activity. You are on your way to a leaner, healthier body. Try a variety of activities such as biking, power-walking, aerobic class or videos, etc. Maybe even consider training for a special event such as a fun-run or walk-a-thon!

For example, "Got up at 6:20 am, dressed, and drank two cups of coffee with cream and sugar. Then I made breakfast for the kids—pancakes and eggs. I ate three bites of my son's leftover pancake, with syrup and butter. I washed it down with his leftover milk." Continue logging the events of your day in this manner.

Final Phase—and from now on!

If you are seeing and feeling a difference, keep doing what you have been doing! You are ready for the next step, the "3 Apple-a-Day" Plan. You have laid your foundation and will continue to make progress. Once you have reached your goal, you'll want to switch to a maintenance program.

In your maintenance program, your food choices will be the same, but you will need to increase your calories so you can maintain *your* ideal weight, and not continue to lose more. Activity can remain the same.

FAQ's for the "3 Apple-a-Day" Plan

1. What is the "3 Apple-a-Day" Plan?

Originally, it was a simple suggestion of eating an apple before each major meal to increase produce consumption and fiber. Later, it was combined with a balanced meal plan that has proven successful for thousands in achieving permanent fat loss.

2. How do apples work in fat loss?

There are several ways the apples aid in fat loss. Apples are not only packed with essential vitamins and minerals, they also provide a high amount of fiber and, when eaten prior to a meal, can help fill you up so you will eat less. Apples are crunchy and sweet and help curb the "sweet tooth." Apples are also very convenient to carry with you. If you're traveling in the car, they are a handy snack to tide you over until you can eat a meal. This will prevent you from making unhealthy quick stop choices.

3. Can other fruits, apple juice or applesauce be substituted?

We feature apples not only because of their convenience, but also because of their nutrient value and low glycemic ranking. Not many fruits can measure up to what apples provide. In the original food plan, there were other fruits listed, with only one apple per day. It wasn't until we started suggesting three apples per day, prior to the meal that we started seeing record fat loss numbers in our local "Get-in-Shape" contest.

4. Why is it so difficult to lose weight when it used to be so easy?

It all depends on how you lost weight in the past. If you lost weight by cutting your calories way down, as most people do, and not exercising, then you probably lost some muscle tissue along the way. Muscle tissue is what keeps metabolism high and, in turn, keeps body fat low. In addition, as you age, if you don't use your muscle you'll lose it (it shrinks) resulting in an even lower metabolism. So in a nutshell, yo-yo dieting strips away your muscle tissue, hangs on to your fat, and makes it extremely difficult to lose weight as you get older.

5. My friend and I weigh the same, but she can wear two sizes smaller.

Your friend likely has a lower body fat and higher muscle tissue ratio than you do. Muscle is much heavier than fat, but takes up a lot less space.

6. Why does it seem easier for men to lose weight faster than women?

Men normally have higher metabolic rates due to higher muscle mass compared to women. The more muscle tissue you have, the more calories you'll burn. So ladies, you can speed up your fat loss by increasing your muscle—through weight training.

7. I have a hard time drinking water. Why is it necessary?

Water has many functions. The most important functions in fat loss are keeping the kidneys flushed and carrying water-soluble vitamins. Also, a high volume of water keeps you feeling full.

8. Why are high-protein, low-carb diets so popular?

They seem to be popular because of the quick weight loss effect. Our society wants instant gratification and this type of diet may show that. Be careful, though. These diets are difficult to stick with long term and may be too low in fiber for a healthy gut. Make sure you are eating 5-9 servings of fruits and vegetables every day on this type of diet.

9. Why do they say "diets don't work"?

Diet alone is not enough to permanently change your metabolism. "Diets" are usually a quick fix and are strongly associated with deprivation. Many diets set people up for temporary weight loss but are often too restrictive or complicated to follow long term. People end up getting frustrated, or have difficulty seeing results and stop doing the diet.

10. What is the difference between "good" fats and "bad" fats?

Good" fats, such as unsaturated (plant oils, fish oil, nuts) are associated with health and prevention of diseases. "Bad" fats, such as trans fats and saturated fats, are just the opposite—associated with disease. In fat loss, fat is fat. It is not very metabolically active and it doesn't take much effort to store excess dietary fat. The "3 Apple-a-Day" Plan recommends your fat intake around 20% of your calories. When you consume fat, try to make sure it's from an unsaturated source and in its original form (i.e. flaxseeds versus flaxseed oil).

11. How can I avoid losing muscle tissue when I'm on a weight loss program?

There are two things that will help: 1) Make sure you are eating enough calories—starting with 10 calories per pound body weight; 2) Weight training will stress the muscle and make it more metabolically active.

12. What's this I hear a lot about "good" and "bad" carbs?

"Good" or "bad" carbs may be termed that in their rating on the Glycemic Index. Good carbs would have a low number, such as apples. A bad carb, such as white bread or refined foods would have a high number. In a simple terms, when carbs have a high glycemic rating, and are eaten alone (not combined with a low glycemic food) they tend to be easily stored as fat, thus making us even fatter.

PART VI

Meal Plans and Recipes

1200-2500 Calorie Daily Plans

Shopping List

Substitution List

Recipes

Eating and cooking with the "3 Apple-a-Day" Plan

The "3 Apple-a-Day" Plan features seven days of planned meals tailored to your specific needs (one diet does not fit all, remember?) There are six levels starting at 1200 up to 2500 calories.

The breakfast contains high fiber carbohydrates and protein to raise and maintain your energy levels through the day. At the end of the day—your last meal—is higher in protein and lower in carbohydrates to allow your body to rest at night. Once you reach your goal and are ready for maintenance, then you can add more carbohydrates to your evening meal. But for now, keep it "light at night."

Refer to the Nutrient Chart in Chapter 11 to determine your starting calorie and nutrient levels.

Over 100 delicious recipes to choose from!

You will not feel deprived on the "3 Apple-a-Day" Plan. You will find satisfying main courses, delicious entrees, hearty breakfast items, healthy snacks and much more. Each recipe provides a per-serving breakdown of calories, protein, carbohydrate, fat, fiber and sodium.

That means you won't have to wonder at the end of the day if you consumed your 40/40/20 (40 percent protein, 40 percent carbohydrates, 20 percent fat) recommendation. Or if you spiked your blood sugar into orbit with high glycemic foods that went right to your hips—since almost all the recipes in the meal plans are comprised of low glycemic ingredients. Some of the meal plans will vary in protein, carbohydrates and fat from the 40/40/20.

The recipes are marked with an asterisk (*). Because calories levels vary, make sure you check your menu recipes to see if there is additional serving suggestions or additions to your recipe. It will follow the listed recipe on the menu.

Glycemic Index ranges

In the substitution list, most of the carbohydrate containing foods have a listed GI number (refer to the Glycemic ratings in Chapter 7).

Variety is the spice of life. Or not!

If you like variety in your meals, there are seven different plans to satisfy those fickle taste buds. If your daily routine is busy and you prefer the simplicity of following the same one-day meal plan throughout the week, that's perfectly acceptable, too.

For added interest, you may even want to mix and match the meals or days and utilize the substitution list. The Sunday "brunch" will also add variety and excitement.

Create your own daily meal

You also have the option of creating your own meal plan. Simply use the guide located next to day one titled "Create your own." This takes more planning, of course, but you will benefit from learning how to balance your own food and make healthier choices.

Create your own recipes

Eating healthy doesn't have to be bland and boring. You can create your own tasty, exciting recipes from your own favorites, many of which can be changed to create a healthier meal. So you don't have to give up the foods you love. Several of the recipes that follow were created by people who have followed the Plan.

Simply exchange some of the less healthy items in your recipes, such as oils and saturated fats, with items and foods found in the substitution list. It not only will be healthier, it will be adventurous!

Who ever said playing with your food was a bad thing?

How to use the substitution list

First, find the food you want to replace in the meal plan. Then find it listed in the substitution list and make an exchange with another preferred choice within that category. For example, if you do not eat beef, exchange the same quantity (try to match the calories and protein) for chicken breast (or whatever you like).

Other healthy tips to boost nutrition:

Item	Instead of...	Try...
Coffee	Cream & sugar	Skim milk and protein powder
In baked goods;	Butter & oil	Applesauce, applebutter
	White flour	Use 1/2 whole wheat
	Quick oatmeal	Old-fashioned oats
	Sugar	Sugar substitute
	Full amount of nuts	Cut it in half
Dairy products	Full-fat	low-fat or skim
	Whole egg	2 egg whites or 1/4 cup egg sub.
Stir-fry or saute'	Oil	Cooking spray or broth
Salad dressing	Regular, full fat	Light or nonfat
Meats	Regular ground beef	7 percent fat or Less

Meal Plans

* Represents the recipes in the Meal Plans

1200 Calorie Meal Plan

Create your own

Breakfast
Protein - 20 grams
Carbohydrate - 30 grams
Fat - 5 grams

Snack
Protein - 20 grams
Carbohydrates - 25 grams

Lunch
Vegetable
Protein - 30 grams
Carbohydrates - 30 grams
Fat - 5 grams

Snack
Protein - 20 grams
Carbohydrates - 25 grams

Dinner
Carbohydrates - 20 grams
Vegetables x 2
Protein - 30 grams
Fat - 5 grams

Calories: 1200
Protein: 120 grams (40%)
Carbs: 120 grams (40%)
Fat: 27 grams (20%)
Fiber: 25 grams
Sodium: 2000 mg

Day 1

Breakfast
Apple
Scrambled Eggs with Salsa*
1/2 cup old-fashioned cooked oatmeal

Snack
1 cup nonfat cottage cheese

Lunch
Apple
1 Sizzlin' Chicken Breast*
1 cup steamed broccoli
1/4 cup Tasty Brown Rice*

Snack
Cappuccino Shake*

Dinner
Grilled Salmon Salad*

Calories: 1235
Protein: 128 grams (41%)
Carbs: 128 grams (41%)
Fat: 23 grams (17%)
Fiber: 23 grams
Sodium: 2349 mg

Recipe found in recipe section

Note: Carbs = Carbohydrates

1200 Calorie Meal Plan

Day 2

Breakfast
Apple
Cheese Omelet*

Snack
8 ounces nonfat yogurt

Lunch
Apple
Turkey Salsa Burger*
1 ounce nonfat sliced cheese
1 cup steamed asparagus

Snack
Strawberry Shake*

Dinner
Apple
Chicken-Broccoli Salad*

Calories: 1205
Protein: 116 grams (39%)
Carbs: 140 grams (45%)
Fat: 22 grams (16%)
Fiber: 25 grams
Sodium: 2733 mg

Day 3

Breakfast
Gourmet Oatmeal*

Snack
Banana Strawberry Smoothie*
1/2 serving

Lunch
Apple
Turkey Lasagna* 1 serving
2 cups tossed green salad
2 tablespoons nonfat dressing

Snack
Mocha Shake*

Dinner
Chicken-Apple Stir-fry*
1 serving

Calories: 1248
Protein: 113 grams (35%)
Carbs: 187 grams (58%)
Fat: 9 grams (7%)
Fiber: 33 grams
Sodium: 1605 mg

Recipe found in recipe section

Note: Carbs = Carbohydrates

1200 Calorie Meal Plan

Day 4

Breakfast
Apple
3/4 cup high-fiber cereal
1/2 cup skim milk

Snack
1 celery stalk
1 tablespoon peanut butter

Lunch
Apple
Beef Stew* 1 serving

Snack
Banana Cream Shake*

Dinner
Apple
Tuna Mixed Green Salad*

Calories: 1229
Protein: 114 grams (36%)
Carbs: 164grams (52%)
Fat: 16 grams (12%)
Fiber: 32 grams
Sodium: 1627 mg

Day 5

Breakfast
Apple
Cheesy Asparagus Omelet*

Snack
Cottage Cheese Yogurt*

Lunch
Apple
Spaghetti Sauce* 1 serving
1/2 cup whole-wheat pasta

Snack
Chocolate Shake*

Dinner
Apple
Salmon Caesar Salad*

Calories: 1209
Protein: 116 grams (38%)
Carbs: 138 grams (46%)
Fat: 22 grams (16%)
Fiber: 22 grams
Sodium: 2419 mg

*Recipe found in recipe section

Note: Carbs = Carbohydrates

1200 Calorie Meal Plan

Day 6

Breakfast
Apple
Tortilla & Eggs*

Snack
8 ounces nonfat yogurt

Lunch
Apple
Hearty Chili* 1 serving

Snack
Strawberry-Banana Shake*

Dinner
Waldorf Salad*

Calories: 1304
Protein: 119 grams (36%)
Carbs: 180 grams (54%)
Fat: 15 grams (10%)
Fiber: 27 grams
Sodium: 2630 mg

Day 7

Breakfast-Brunch
Apple slices
Fat-free Cinnamon Roll*
2 Deviled Eggs*

Snack
Salmon Crackers*

Lunch
Apple
Turkey Rice Mix* 1 serving
1 cup broccoli

Snack
French Vanilla Shake*

Dinner
Taco Salad* 1 serving

Dessert
Mock Apple Pie* 1 serving

Calories: 1349
Protein: 114 grams (34%)
Carbs: 187 grams (56%)
Fat: 16 grams (10%)
Fiber: 26 grams
Sodium: 1020 mg

Recipe found in recipe section

Note: Carbs = Carbohydrates

1500 Calorie Meal Plan

Create your own

Breakfast
Protein - 30 grams
Carbohydrates - 30 grams
Fat - 8 grams

Snack
Protein - 30 grams
Carbohydrates - 30 grams

Lunch
Vegetable
Protein - 30 grams
Carbohydrates - 40 grams
Fat - 8 grams

Snack
Protein - 30 grams
Carbohydrates - 30 grams

Dinner
Carbohydrates - 20 grams
Vegetables x 2
Protein - 30 grams
Fat - 8 grams

Calories: 1500
Protein: 150 grams (40%)
Carbs: 150 grams (40%)
Fat: 33 grams (20%)
Fiber: 25 grams
Sodium: 2000 mg

Day 1

Breakfast
Apple
Scrambled Eggs with Salsa*
1 cup old-fashioned cooked oatmeal

Snack
1 cup nonfat cottage cheese

Lunch
Apple
1 Sizzlin' Chicken Breast*
1 cup steamed broccoli
1/4 cup Tasty Brown Rice*

Snack
Cappuccino Shake*

Dinner
Grilled Salmon Salad*
(6 ounces salmon)

Calories: 1570
Protein: 158 grams (40%)
Carbs: 156 grams (40%)
Fat: 35 grams (20%)
Fiber: 26 grams
Sodium: 2751 mg

Recipe found in recipe section

Note: Carbs = Carbohydrates

1500 Calorie Meal Plan

Day 2

Breakfast
Apple
Ham & Cheese Omelet*

Snack
8 ounces nonfat yogurt

Lunch
Apple
Turkey Salsa Burger*
1 ounce nonfat sliced cheese
1 cup steamed asparagus

Snack
Strawberry Shake*

Dinner
Apple
Chicken-Broccoli Salad*

Calories: 1498
Protein: 178 grams (46%)
Carbs: 140 grams (37%)
Fat: 28 grams (17%)
Fiber: 25 grams
Sodium: 3643 mg

Day 3

Breakfast
Gourmet Oatmeal*

Snack
Banana Strawberry Smoothie*

Lunch
Apple
Turkey Lasagna* 1 serving
2 cups tossed green salad
2 tablespoons nonfat dressing

Snack
Mocha Shake*

Dinner
Chicken-Apple Stir-fry*
1 serving

Calories: 1510
Protein: 124 grams (32%)
Carbs: 232 grams (59%)
Fat: 15 grams (9%)
Fiber: 40 grams
Sodium: 1700 mg

*Recipe found in recipe section

Note: Carbs = Carbohydrates

1500 Calorie Meal Plan

Day 4

Breakfast
Apple
3/4 cup high-fiber cereal
1/2 cup skim milk

Snack
1 celery stalk
2 tablespoons peanut butter

Lunch
Apple
Beef Stew* 1 serving

Snack
Banana Cream Shake*

Dinner
Apple
Tuna Mixed Green Salad*

Calories: 1497
Protein: 145 grams (38%)
Carbs: 179 grams (47%)
Fat: 24 grams (15%)
Fiber: 34 grams
Sodium: 1760 mg

Day 5

Breakfast
Apple
Cheesy Asparagus Omelet*
(double the cheese)

Snack
Cottage Cheese Yogurt*

Lunch
Apple
Spaghetti Sauce* 1 serving
1/2 cup whole-wheat pasta

Snack
Chocolate Shake*

Dinner
Apple
Salmon Caesar Salad*
(6 ounces salmon)

Calories: 1463
Protein: 149 grams (41%)
Carbs: 144 grams (39%)
Fat: 33 grams (20%)
Fiber: 22 grams
Sodium: 3150 mg

*Recipe found in recipe section

Note: Carbs = Carbohydrates

1500 Calorie Meal Plan

Day 6

Breakfast
Apple
Tortilla & Eggs*

Snack
8 ounces nonfat yogurt

Lunch
Apple
Hearty Chili* 1 serving

Snack
Strawberry-Banana Shake*

Dinner
Waldorf Salad*
(double chicken & nuts)

Calories: 1536
Protein: 148 grams (38%)
Carbs: 187 grams (48%)
Fat: 25 grams (14%)
Fiber: 29 grams
Sodium: 2891 mg

Day 7

Breakfast-Brunch
Apple slices
Fat-free Cinnamon Roll*
3 Deviled Eggs*

Snack
Salmon Crackers*
(2 ounces salmon)

Lunch
Apple
Turkey Rice Mix* 1 serving
1 cup broccoli

Snack
French Vanilla Shake*

Dinner
Taco Salad* 1 serving

Dessert
Mock Apple Pie* 1 serving

Calories: 1498
Protein: 133 grams (36%)
Carbs: 188 grams (50%)
Fat: 23 grams (14%)
Fiber: 26 grams
Sodium: 1186 mg

*Recipe found in recipe section

Note: Carbs = Carbohydrates

1800 Calorie Meal Plan

Create your own

Breakfast
Protein - 36 grams
Carbohydrate - 40 grams
Fat - 10 grams

Snack
Protein - 36 grams
Carbohydrates - 40 grams

Lunch
Vegetable
Protein - 36 grams
Carbohydrates - 40 grams
Fat - 10 grams

Snack
Protein - 36 grams
Carbohydrates - 40 grams

Dinner
Carbohydrates - 20 grams
Vegetables x 2
Protein - 36 grams
Fat - 10 grams

Calories: 1800
Protein: 180 grams (40%)
Carbs: 180 grams (40%)
Fat: 40 grams (20%)
Fiber: 30 grams
Sodium: 2500 mg

Day 1

Breakfast
Apple
Scrambled Eggs with Salsa*
1 cup old-fashioned cooked oatmeal

Snack
1 cup nonfat cottage cheese

Lunch
Apple
1-1/2 Sizzlin' Chicken Breast*
1 cup steamed broccoli
1 cup Tasty Brown Rice*

Snack
Cappuccino Shake*

Dinner
Grilled Salmon Salad*
(6 ounces salmon)

Calories: 1824
Protein: 186 grams (41%)
Carbs: 181 grams (40%)
Fat: 38 grams (19%)
Fiber: 28 grams
Sodium: 3285 mg

Recipe found in recipe section

Note: Carbs = Carbohydrates

1800 Calorie Meal Plan

Day 2

Breakfast
Apple
Ham & Cheese Omelet*

Snack
8 ounces nonfat yogurt

Lunch
Apple
Turkey Salsa Burger*
on a whole wheat kaiser bun
1 ounce nonfat sliced cheese
1 cup steamed asparagus

Snack
Strawberry Shake*

Dinner
Apple
Chicken-Broccoli Salad*
(6 ounces chicken breast)

Calories: 1791
Protein: 213 grams (46%)
Carbs: 170 grams (37%)
Fat: 33 grams (17%)
Fiber: 31 grams
Sodium: 4580 mg

Day 3

Breakfast
Gourmet Oatmeal*

Snack
Banana Strawberry Smoothie*

Lunch
Apple
Turkey Lasagna* 1-1/2serving
2 cups tossed green salad
2 tablespoons nonfat dressing

Snack
Mocha Shake*

Dinner
Chicken-Apple Stir-fry*
2 servings

Calories: 1832
Protein: 168 grams (36%)
Carbs: 260 grams (55%)
Fat: 19 grams (9%)
Fiber: 46 grams
Sodium: 2363 mg

*Recipe found in recipe section

Note: Carbs = Carbohydrates

1800 Calorie Meal Plan

Day 4

Breakfast
Apple
1-1/2 cups high-fiber cereal
1 cup skim milk

Snack
1 celery stalk
2 tablespoons peanut butter

Lunch
Apple
Beef Stew* 2 servings

Snack
Banana Cream Shake Deluxe*

Dinner
Apple
Tuna Mixed Green Salad*

Calories: 1791
Protein: 172 grams (38%)
Carbs: 218 grams (47%)
Fat: 28 grams (15%)
Fiber: 41 grams
Sodium: 2237 mg

Day 5

Breakfast
Apple
Cheesy Asparagus Omelet*
(double the cheese)

Snack
Cottage Cheese Yogurt*
1-1/2 servings

Lunch
Apple
Spaghetti Sauce* 2 servings
1 cup whole-wheat pasta

Snack
Chocolate Shake*

Dinner
Apple
Salmon Caesar Salad*
(6 ounces salmon)

Calories: 1795
Protein: 180 grams (40%)
Carbs: 178 grams (40%)
Fat: 40 grams (20%)
Fiber: 29 grams
Sodium: 3850 mg

*Recipe found in recipe section

Note: Carbs = Carbohydrates

1800 Calorie Meal Plan

Day 6

Breakfast
Apple
Tortilla & Eggs*
2 servings

Snack
Blueberry Peach Smoothie*

Lunch
Apple
Hearty Chili* 1 serving

Snack
Strawberry-Banana Shake*

Dinner
Waldorf Salad*
(double chicken & nuts)

Calories: 1803
Protein: 160 grams (35%)
Carbs: 231 grams (50%)
Fat: 31 grams (15%)
Fiber: 39 grams
Sodium: 3061 mg

Day 7

Breakfast-Brunch
Apple slices
Fat-free Cinnamon Roll*
6 Deviled Eggs*

Snack
Salmon Crackers*
(2 ounces salmon)

Lunch
Apple
Turkey Rice Mix* 1 serving
1 cup broccoli

Snack
French Vanilla Shake*

Dinner
Taco Salad* 2 servings

Dessert
Mock Apple Pie* 1 serving

Calories: 1794
Protein: 175 grams (39%)
Carbs: 196 grams (44%)
Fat: 34 grams (17%)
Fiber: 28 grams
Sodium: 1694 mg

*Recipe found in recipe section

Note: Carbs = Carbohydrates

2000 Calorie Meal Plan

Create your own

Breakfast
Protein - 40 grams
Carbohydrate - 50 grams
Fat - 12 grams

Snack
Protein - 40 grams
Carbohydrates - 40 grams

Lunch
Vegetable
Protein - 40 grams
Carbohydrates - 50 grams
Fat - 12 grams

Snack
Protein - 40 grams
Carbohydrates - 40 grams

Dinner
Carbohydrates - 20 grams
Vegetables x 2
Protein - 36 grams
Fat - 12 grams

Calories: 2000
Protein: 200 grams (40%)
Carbs: 200 grams (40%)
Fat: 44 grams (20%)
Fiber: 35 grams
Sodium: 3000 mg

Day 1

Breakfast
Apple
Scrambled Eggs with Salsa*
1 cup old-fashioned cooked oatmeal

Snack
1 cup nonfat cottage cheese

Lunch
Apple
1-1/2 Sizzlin' Chicken Breast*
1 cup steamed broccoli
1 cup Tasty Brown Rice*

Snack
Peanut Butter Shake Deluxe*

Dinner
Grilled Salmon Salad*
(6 ounces salmon)

Calories: 2002
Protein: 191 grams (38%)
Carbs: 205 grams (41%)
Fat: 47 grams (21%)
Fiber: 32 grams
Sodium: 3388 mg

*Recipe found in recipe section

Note: Carbs = Carbohydrates

2000 Calorie Meal Plan

Day 2

Breakfast
Apple
Ham & Cheese Omelet*

Snack
8 ounces nonfat yogurt
1/2 cup lowfat granola

Lunch
Apple
2 Turkey Salsa Burgers*
on a whole wheat kaiser bun
1 ounce nonfat sliced cheese
1 cup steamed asparagus

Snack
Strawberry Shake*

Dinner
Apple
Chicken-Broccoli Salad*
(6 ounces chicken breast)

Calories: 1960
Protein: 219 grams (44%)
Carbs: 205 grams (41%)
Fat: 35 grams (15%)
Fiber: 37 grams
Sodium: 4764 mg

Day 3

Breakfast
Gourmet Oatmeal*
1-1/2 servings

Snack
Banana Strawberry Smoothie*

Lunch
Apple
Turkey Lasagna* 1-1/2serving
2 cups tossed green salad
2 tablespoons nonfat dressing

Snack
Mocha Shake Deluxe*

Dinner
Chicken-Apple Stir-fry*
2 servings

Calories: 1966
Protein: 182 grams (36%)
Carbs: 278 grams (55%)
Fat: 20 grams (9%)
Fiber: 49 grams
Sodium: 2400 mg

Recipe found in recipe section

Note: Carbs = Carbohydrates

2000 Calorie Meal Plan

Day 4

Breakfast
Apple
1-1/2 cups high-fiber cereal
1-1/2 cups skim milk

Snack
1 celery stalk
2 tablespoons peanut butter

Lunch
Apple
Beef Stew* 2 servings

Snack
Banana Cream Shake Deluxe*

Dinner
Apple
Tuna Mixed Green Salad*
(9 ounces tuna)

Calories: 2021
Protein: 202 grams (39%)
Carbs: 232 grams (45%)
Fat: 36 grams (16%)
Fiber: 45 grams
Sodium: 2793 mg

Day 5

Breakfast
Apple
Cheesy Asparagus Omelet*
(double the cheese)

Snack
Cottage Cheese Yogurt*
2 servings

Lunch
Apple
Spaghetti Sauce* 2 servings
1 1/2 cups whole-wheat pasta

Snack
Chocolate Shake Deluxe*

Dinner
Apple
Salmon Caesar Salad*
(6 ounces salmon)

Calories: 1961
Protein: 196 grams (40%)
Carbs: 204 grams (41%)
Fat: 42 grams (19%)
Fiber: 32 grams
Sodium: 4293 mg

*Recipe found in recipe section   Note: Carbs = Carbohydrates

2000 Calorie Meal Plan

Day 6

Breakfast
Apple
Tortilla & Eggs*
2 servings

Snack
Blueberry Peach Smoothie*

Lunch
Apple
Hearty Chili* 2 servings

Snack
Strawberry-Banana Shake*

Dinner
Waldorf Salad*
(double chicken & nuts)

Calories: 2017
Protein: 181 grams (35%)
Carbs: 263 grams (51%)
Fat: 33 grams (14%)
Fiber: 48 grams
Sodium: 3899 mg

Day 7

Breakfast-Brunch
Apple slices
Fat-free Cinnamon Roll*
6 Deviled Eggs*

Snack
Salmon Crackers*
(3 ounces salmon
+2 ounces cream cheese)

Lunch
Apple
Turkey Rice Mix* 1-1/2 servings
1 cup broccoli

Snack
French Vanilla Shake*

Dinner
Taco Salad* 2 servings

Dessert
Mock Apple Pie* 1 serving

Calories: 2017
Protein: 199 grams (40%)
Carbs: 215 grams (43%)
Fat: 39 grams (17%)
Fiber: 28 grams
Sodium: 1870 mg

*Recipe found in recipe section

Note: Carbs = Carbohydrates

2500 Calorie Meal Plan

Create your own

Breakfast
Protein - 50 grams
Carbohydrate - 60 grams
Fat - 14 grams

Snack
Protein - 50 grams
Carbohydrates - 50 grams

Lunch
Vegetable
Protein - 50 grams
Carbohydrates - 70 grams
Fat - 14 grams

Snack
Protein - 50 grams
Carbohydrates - 50 grams

Dinner
Carbohydrates - 20 grams
Vegetables x 2
Protein - 50 grams
Fat - 14 grams

Calories: 2500
Protein: 250 grams (40%)
Carbs: 250 grams (40%)
Fat: 56 grams (20%)
Fiber: 40 grams
Sodium: 3000 mg

*Recipe found in recipe section

Day 1

Breakfast
Apple
Scrambled Eggs with Salsa*
1-1/2 servings
1-1/2 cups old-fashioned
cooked oatmeal

Snack
1 cup nonfat cottage cheese
1 medium pear

Lunch
Apple
2 Sizzlin' Chicken Breast*
1 cup steamed broccoli
1-1/2 cups Tasty Brown Rice*

Snack
Peanut Butter Shake Deluxe*

Dinner
Grilled Salmon Salad*
(6 ounces salmon)

Calories: 2488
Protein: 240 grams (39%)
Carbs: 250 grams (40%)
Fat: 59 grams (21%)
Fiber: 37 grams
Sodium: 4248 mg

Note: Carbs = Carbohydrates

2500 Calorie Meal Plan

Day 2

Breakfast
Apple
2 Ham & Cheese Omelets*

Snack
8 ounces nonfat yogurt
3/4 cup lowfat granola

Lunch
Apple
2 Turkey Salsa Burgers*
on a whole wheat kaiser bun
1 ounce nonfat sliced cheese
1 cup steamed asparagus

Snack
Strawberry Shake*

Dinner
Apple
Chicken-Broccoli Salad*
(6 ounces chicken breast)

Calories: 2456
Protein: 288 grams (46%)
Carbs: 229 grams (37%)
Fat: 48 grams (17%)
Fiber: 41 grams
Sodium: 6956 mg

Day 3

Breakfast
Gourmet Oatmeal*
2 servings

Snack
Banana Strawberry Smoothie*

Lunch
Apple
Turkey Lasagna* 1-1/2servings
3 cups tossed green salad
3 tablespoons nonfat dressing
2 tablespoons sliced almonds

Snack
Mocha Shake Deluxe*

Dinner
Chicken-Apple Stir-fry*
2 servings

Calories: 2492
Protein: 234 grams (37%)
Carbs: 332 grams (52%)
Fat: 31 grams (11%)
Fiber: 57 grams
Sodium: 3095 mg

*Recipe found in recipe section

Note: Carbs = Carbohydrates

2500 Calorie Meal Plan

Day 4

Breakfast
Apple
2 cups high-fiber cereal
1-1/2 cups skim milk

Snack
1 celery stalk
2 tablespoons peanut butter

Lunch
Apple
Beef Stew* 3 servings

Snack
Banana Cream Shake Deluxe*

Dinner
Apple
Tuna Mixed Green Salad*
(12 ounces tuna)

Calories: 2476
Protein: 252 grams (40%)
Carbs: 285 grams (45%)
Fat: 41 grams (15%)
Fiber: 53 grams
Sodium: 3558 mg

Day 5

Breakfast
Apple
2 Cheesy Asparagus Omelet*

Snack
Cottage Cheese Yogurt*
2 servings

Lunch
Apple
Spaghetti Sauce* 2 servings
1-1/2 cups whole-wheat pasta

Snack
Chocolate Shake Deluxe*

Dinner
Apple
Salmon Caesar Salad*
(9 ounces salmon)

Calories: 2479
Protein: 262 grams (43%)
Carbs: 223 grams (36%)
Fat: 58 grams (21%)
Fiber: 33 grams
Sodium: 4916 mg

*Recipe found in recipe section

Note: Carbs = Carbohydrates

2500 Calorie Meal Plan

Day 6

Breakfast
Apple
Tortilla & Eggs*
2 servings
(add 2 ounces nonfat cheese)

Snack
Blueberry Peach Smoothie*

Lunch
Apple
Hearty Chili* 2 servings

Snack
Strawberry-Banana Shake Deluxe*

Dinner
Waldorf Salad*
(double chicken & nuts)

Calories: 2505
Protein: 239 grams (37%)
Carbs: 310 grams (48%)
Fat: 42 grams (15%)
Fiber: 51 grams
Sodium: 4325 mg

Day 7

Breakfast-Brunch
Apple slices
Fat-free Cinnamon Roll*
6 Deviled Eggs*

Snack
Salmon Crackers*
(3 ounces salmon
+ 2 ounces cream cheese)

Lunch
Apple
Turkey Rice Mix* 2 servings
1 cup broccoli

Snack
French Vanilla Shake Deluxe*

Dinner
Taco Salad* 2 servings

Dessert
Mock Apple Pie* 1 serving

Calories: 2515
Protein: 249 grams (40%)
Carbs: 278 grams (45%)
Fat: 40 grams (15%)
Fiber: 35 grams
Sodium: 2147 mg

*Recipe found in recipe section

Note: Carbs = Carbohydrates

3 APPLE-A-DAY SHOPPING LIST

Weekly Groceries

Meats, fish and poultry
Chicken breast
Turkey breast
4% lean ground beef
Flank steak
Salmon

Vegetables, fresh
Broccoli
Cauliflower
Onion
Mushrooms
Lettuce, romaine & mixed
Spinach
Asparagus
Zucchini
Green and red peppers
Celery
Carrot
Red potatoes
Tomato
Sugar snap peas
Bean sprouts

Fruits, fresh
Apples
Strawberries
Banana
Blueberries
Peaches

Eggs and dairy
Skim milk
Nonfat cottage cheese
Nonfat yogurt
Eggs
Egg substitute
Nonfat shredded cheddar cheese
Nonfat shredded mozzarella cheese
Nonfat sliced cheese
Nonfat cream cheese
Parmesan cheese, shredded
Light margarine

Canned goods
Tuna, Albacore
Chicken breast
Salmon
Kidney beans, low sodium
Black beans
Italian stewed tomatoes, diced
Tomato paste
Tomato sauce
Evaporated skim milk

Grains and cereals
Oatmeal, regular old-fashioned
High fiber cereal, low sodium
Spaghetti noodles, whole wheat
Lasagna noodles
Brown or wild rice
Flour tortilla, whole wheat
Rye crisp crackers, fat free
Low-fat granola

Pantry Staples

Herbs and spices
Cinnamon
Garlic powder
Basil
Oregano
Chili powder
Salt
Pepper
Taco seasoning

Other items
Chicken bouillon cubes
Peanut butter, reduced-fat
Coffee
Whole wheat Kaiser rolls
Protein powder (soy or whey)

Baking goods
Whole wheat flour
Enriched white flour
Sugar
Sugar substitute (Splenda™)
Yeast
Applesauce, unsweetened
Raisins
Walnuts, almonds
Brown sugar
Powdered sugar
Vanilla extract

Condiments
Salsa
Rice vinegar
Soy sauce, low sodium
Salad dressings, nonfat or light
Dijon mustard
Fat free liquid coffee creamer, French Vanilla
Worcestershire sauce
Teriyaki sauce
Nonfat mayonnaise

This shopping list is only for the foods and recipe items in the seven-day meal plans. If you are using other recipes, make sure you add the additional food ingredients to your weekly shopping list.

SUBSTITUTION LIST

Use this substitution list by replacing foods in the meal plan that are within the same group. For example: in the Proteins, replace three ounces of salmon for three ounces of chicken breast.

	Amount	Calories	Protein(g)	Carbs(g)	Fat(g)	Fiber(g)	GI	omega 6	omega 3
Proteins									
Chicken breast	3 ounces	140	26	0	3	0	-	0.4	Trace
Turkey breast	3 ounces	114	26	0	0.6	0	-	0.27	0.01
Extra lean beef	3 ounces	201	26	0	10	0	-	0.3	Trace
Tuna	3 ounces	99	22	0	0.7	0	-	0.3	0.3
Halibut, Bass, Snapper	3 ounces	119	23	0	2.5	0	-	0.2	0.1
Salmon	3 ounces	155	22	0	7	0	-	0.6	0.1
Cod, Orange Roughy	3 ounces	89	20	0	0.7	0	-	Trace	Trace
Shrimp	3 ounces	118	23	1	1.9	0	-	0.1	Trace
Skim milk	1 cup	80	8	11	1	0	32	0.1	0.005
Nonfat cottage cheese	1 cup	121	25	3	0.6	0	-	-	-
Nonfat yogurt	1 cup	127	13	17	0.4	0	14	-	-
Egg whites, egg substitute	6, 1 cup	99	21	2	0	0	-	-	-
Kidney beans/legumes	3/4 cup	163	11	29	0.6	7	27	0.3	0.6
Light tofu	332 grams	124	21	4	2.7	0	-	0.14	0.22
Vegetable burger	113 grams	200	10	28	5	4	-	2.3	0.14
Whey protein powder	5 Tbls.	115	20	4	2	1	-	-	-
Carbohydrates / Grains									
Regular oatmeal, cooked	1 cup	145	6	25	2.3	5	49	0.39	0.34
Whole wheat hot cereal	1 cup	133	5	28	1	4	-	-	-
Potato, baked	202 grams	220	5	51	0.2	5	85	0.65	0.02
Sweet potato, yam	1 cup	158	2	38	0.2	5	54	0.08	0.016
Brown rice	1 cup	232	5	50	1	3	55	-	-
Pasta, whole wheat	1 cup	197	7	40	1	4	37	0.28	0.14
Cereal, Kashi Go-Lean	1 cup	160	11	37	1	13	-	-	-
Cereal, shredded wheat	1 cup	167	5	41	0.5	6	58	-	-
Rye Crisp, fat-free crackers	2 pieces	48	2	10	0	1.5	69	-	-

	Amount	Calories	Protein(g)	Carbs(g)	Fat(g)	Fiber(g)	GI	omega 6	omega 3

Fruit

	Amount	Calories	Protein(g)	Carbs(g)	Fat(g)	Fiber(g)	GI	omega 6	omega 3
Apple, medium	1 each	81	0.3	21	0.5	4	38	0.12	0.025
Banana, small	1 each	93	1	24	0.5	2	55	0.057	0.03
Cherries	10 whole	45	1	10	0	1	22	0.1	0.1
Apricots	3 small	50	1.5	12	0.4	2.5	57	0.081	0
Grapefruit	1 whole	74	1.4	18	0.2	3	25	0.047	0.012
Grapes	1 cup						46	0.07	0.022
Nectarine	1 medium	67	1.3	16	0.6	2	-	0.3	0.007
Orange	1 medium	64	1	16	0	3	44	0.047	0.017
Pear	1 small	98	0.6	25	0.6	4	38	0.15	0.002
Peach	1 medium	42	0.6	11	0	2	42	0.043	0.001

Vegetables - not limited to

	Amount	Calories	Protein(g)	Carbs(g)	Fat(g)	Fiber(g)	GI	omega 6	omega 3
Broccoli, raw	1 cup	27	3	5	0.3	2.5	-	0.03	0.1
Cauliflower, raw	1 cup	28	2	5	0.2	3	-	0.02	0.076
Cabbage, raw	1 cup	33	1.5	7	0.6	3.5	-	0.036	0.048
Mushrooms, raw	1 cup	18	2	3	0.2	1	-	0.128	0.001
Spinach, raw	1 cup	7	1	1	0	1	-	0.007	0.0035
Zucchini, raw	1 cup	29	1	7	0	3	-	0.025	0.042
Asparagus, cooked	1 cup	43	5	8	0	3	-	-	-
Green beans, cooked	1 cup	44	2.4	10	0.3	4	-	0.07	0.11
Carrots, raw baby	10	86	2	18.5	4	1	49	0.34	0.05
Romaine lettuce	1 cup	8	1	1	1	1	-	0.017	0.04
Green leaf lettuce	1 cup	10	0.7	2	1	0	-	0.26	0.01

Fats

	Amount	Calories	Protein(g)	Carbs(g)	Fat(g)	Fiber(g)	GI	omega 6	omega 3
Canola oil	1 Tbls	124	0	0	14	0	-	2.84	1.3
Olive oil	1 Tbls	119	0	0	13.5	0	-	1.067	0.08
Flaxseed oil	1 Tbls	124	0	0	14	0	-	-	-
Flax seeds, whole	1 Tbls	59	2	4	4	3	-	0.5	2.17
Walnuts	1 Tbls	47	2	1	4.4	0.4	-	2.61	0.25

Recipes

❖

Breakfast Foods

Eggs

Shakes

Poultry, Fish and Meat

Main Entrees

Salads & Vegetables

Snacks & Appetizers

Desserts & Sweets

❖

BREAKFAST FOODS

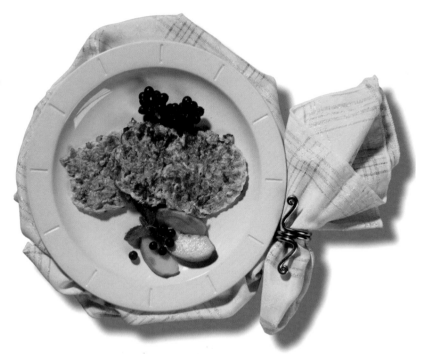

Oat Cakes

<u>Quick</u>

1 cup regular old-fashioned oatmeal,
    uncooked
6 egg whites
1 cup nonfat cottage cheese

Beat egg whites with a fork until bubbly.
Add oats and cottage cheese. Spray a skillet
with nonstick cooking spray and place over
medium heat. Pour 1/4 cup mixture, in
three spots, spacing at least 3 inches apart.
Cook until golden brown. Makes 8.

Optional: Top with nonfat yogurt and
cooked diced apples.

Each cake without topping:

Calories: 61	*Fat: 0.3 grams*
Protein: 7 grams	*Fiber: 1 gram*
Carbohydrates: 8 grams	*Sodium: 114 mg*

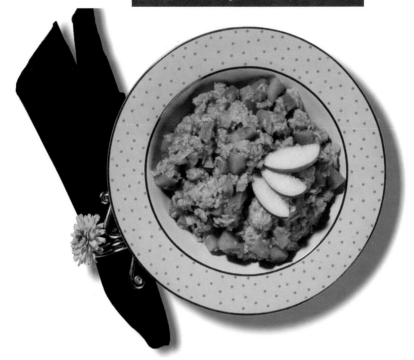

Gourmet Oatmeal

Quick

1 cup cooked oatmeal
1 medium apple
2 tablespoons vanilla protein powder
1 teaspoon cinnamon

Mix all ingredients and enjoy! You can also cook apples with the oatmeal. Serves 1.

Calories: 252   *Fat: 1.5 grams*
Protein: 11 grams   *Fiber: 9 grams*
Carbohydrates: 53 grams   *Sodium: 24 mg*

Cereal Blend

Quick

1 cup high-fiber, low sodium cereal
1/2 cup shredded wheat, spoon size
1/4 cup lowfat granola
1 cup skim milk

Mix cereals and add milk. Serves 1.

Calories: 368   *Fat: 2.8 grams*
Protein: 21 grams   *Fiber: 14 grams*
Carbohydrates: 77 grams   *Sodium: 240 mg*

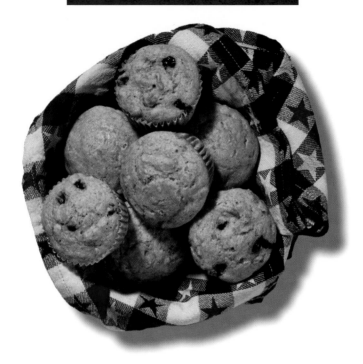

Bran Muffins

3/4 cup flour
1/2 cup whole wheat flour
1 tables~~~ ~~~ king powder
1/2

~~~an cereal
~~~ ~~~ ~~~nilk
2 egg whites
1/4 cup applesauce

Combine flours, baking powder, sugar and salt; set aside. In a mixing bowl, combine cereal and milk; let stand for two minutes. Add egg and applesauce; mix well. Add dry ingredients, stirring just until combined. Spoon into 12 muffin cups coated with nonstick cooking spray. Bake at 400 degrees for 15-18 minutes or until golden brown. Add 1 cup berries for variety. Serve warm. Serves 12.

Calories: 95   *Fat: 0*
Protein: 4 grams   *Fiber: 2.4 grams*
Carbohydrates: 20 grams   *Sodium: 131 mg*

Breakfast Quesadilla

<u>Quick</u>

1/2 cup egg substitute
1 tablespoon green pepper, diced
1 tablespoon onion, chopped
1 ounce nonfat shredded cheddar cheese
2 low-fat whole wheat tortillas
1 ounce nonfat shredded mozzarella
   cheese
2 tablespoons mild salsa

Microwave or use a skillet and cook eggs, pepper, onion and cheddar cheese. Cook flat, and flip once. Heat tortillas in microwave for 30 seconds. Place egg mixture on first tortilla and cover with the second tortilla. Sprinkle with mozarella cheese, and top with salsa. Serves 1.

Calories: 297   *Fat: 1.5 grams*
Protein: 29 grams   *Fiber: 4 grams*
Carbohydrates: 53 grams   *Sodium: 1401 mg*

Breakfast Burrito

<u>Quick</u>

1/2 cup egg beaters
1 whole wheat tortilla
1 tablespoon green and red peppers
Light margarine (optional)

Cook egg beaters and peppers in microwave for 1-2 minutes or in small sautee pan over medium heat until eggs are cooked. Heat tortilla in microwave for 20 seconds. Lightly spread margarine on tortilla, then place eggs down the middle and roll up. Serves 1.

Option: Add nonfat cheese and/or salsa. This will add a few more calories.

Calories: 126   *Fat: 0.5 grams*
Protein: 13 grams   *Fiber: 2 grams*
Carbohydrates: 23 grams   *Sodium: 331 mg*

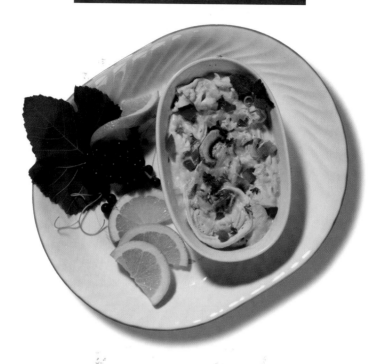

Egg Casserole

Quick

2 cups egg substitute
2 ounces nonfat shredded cheese
8 large mushrooms, sliced
4 tablespoons salsa

Spray microwave safe dish with nonstick
cooking spray. Cook eggs with mushrooms
in microwave until eggs are cooked. Add
cheese and mix. Cook for another 45
seconds until cheese melts. Top with salsa.
Serves 4.

Calories: 87
Protein: 15 grams
Carbohydrates: 6 grams

Fat: 0 gram
Fiber: 0.7 grams
Sodium: 424 mg

Breakfast in a Blender

Quick

6 ounces nonfat milk
5 tablespoons protein powder
 (chocolate or vanilla)
1/2 cup oatmeal, uncooked
1 medium banana
Ice

Blend until smooth.

Calories: 436
Protein: 38 grams
Carbohydrates: 70 grams

Fat: 2 grams
Fiber: 9 grams
Sodium 165 mg

Turkey Breast Sausage Patties *by Rosalie McPherson*

<u>Large Volume Recipe</u>

1/2 cup chopped onion
1/2 cup apple, shredded and peeled
1 garlic clove, minced
3 teaspoons dried thyme
3 teaspoons dried, rubbed sage
1 teaspoon salt
1/2 teaspoon black pepper
2 pounds ground turkey breast
Cooking spray

Heat and spray nonstick cooking spray in skillet over medium-high heat. Add onion and apple; saute' 3 minutes. Add garlic; saute' 30 seconds. Remove onion mixture from pan; cool completely. Combine onion mixture, thyme, sage, salt, pepper, and turkey, stirring well to combine. Divide mixture into 24 equal portions, shaping each into a 1/2 inch thick patty. Heat a large skillet coated with nonstick cooking spray over medium heat. Add half of the patties; cook 3 minutes on each side or until done. Keep warm. Repeat procedure with remaining patties. 8 servings (3 patties per serving).

Calories: 156   *Fat: 3 grams*
Protein: 32 grams   *Fiber: 0 grams*
Carbohydrates: 1 gram   *Sodium: 74 mg*

One-dish Spicy Breakfast Casserole *by Nancy VanHoven*

<u>Quick and Large Volume Recipe</u>

32 ounce can refried beans, fat free
2 tablespoons chili powder
2-4 ounce cans diced green chilies
4 cups egg substitute
1 cup low-fat mozzarella cheese
2 cups salsa

Preheat oven to 350 degrees. Mix chili powder with beans and spread in a 9x13 baking dish. Top with chilies, then pour egg over the chilies. Bake approximately 20-30 minutes, just until the eggs are set. Top with cheese then salsa. Serves 18.

Calories: 76   *Fat: 1.5 grams*
Protein: 6.5 grams   *Fiber: 2.4 grams*
Carbohydrates: 9 grams   *Sodium: 347 mg*

EGGS

Egg White Only Omelet

6 large egg whites
   or 3/4 cup egg substitute
Salsa (optional)

Beat eggs until large bubbles form. Spray small saute pan or omelet pan with non-stick spray. Pour in egg whites and cook over medium heat. Cook egg whites until white and most of the uncooked egg white is cooked. Add the desired ingredients. Fold the egg white circle in half, or just close the omelet pan. Top with salsa and serve. Serves 1.

Calories: 99   *Fat: 0 grams*
Protein: 21 grams   *Fiber: 0 grams*
Carbohydrates: 2 grams *Sodium: 298 mg*

Basic Omelet

1 whole egg
5 egg whites
   or 3/4 cup egg substitute
Salsa (optional)

Beat eggs until large bubbles form. Spray small sauté pan or omelet pan with non-stick spray. Pour in eggs and cook over medium heat. Cook eggs until firm, about 5-6 minutes. Add the desired ingredients. Fold the egg white circle in half, or just close the omelet pan. Top with salsa and serve. Serves 1.

Calories: 188   *Fat: 5 grams*
Protein: 28 grams   *Fiber: 0 grams*
Carbohydrates: 5 grams *Sodium: 411 mg*

Cheese Omelet

Follow directions for Basic Omelet.

Sprinkle 1 ounce nonfat cheddar cheese in the middle.

Calories: 188　　　　*Fat: 5 grams*
Protein: 28 grams　　*Fiber: 0 grams*
Carbohydrates: 5 grams　*Sodium: 411 mg*

Ham & Cheese Omelet

1 ounce extra lean ham
1 ounce cheese
6 large egg whites + 1 yolk

Follow directions for Basic Omelet. Sprinkle the ham and cheese in the middle, then fold the circle in half.

Calories: 225　　　　*Fat: 6.6 grams*
Protein: 34 grams　　*Fiber: 0 grams*
Carbohydrates: 5 grams　*Sodium: 675 mg*

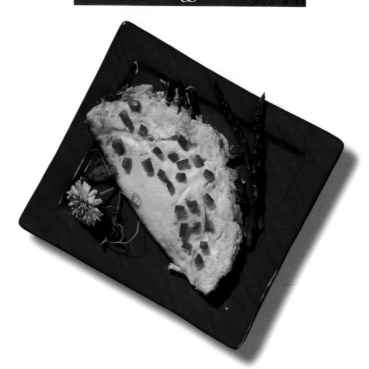

Cheesy Asparagus Omelet

4 small asparagus spears chopped
1 ounce nonfat cheese
6 egg whites + 1 yolk

Follow directions for Basic Omelet. Add asparagus and cheese in the middle, then fold over egg whites.

Calories: 202

Protein: 30 grams

Carbohydrates: 8 grams

Fat: 5 grams

Fiber: 1.3 grams

Sodium: 432 mg

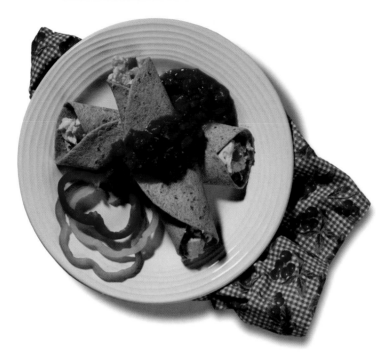

Tortilla & Eggs

1/2 cup egg beaters
1 whole wheat tortilla
1 tablespoon green and red peppers
Light margarine (optional)

Cook egg beaters and peppers in microwave for 1-2 minutes or in small saute' pan over medium heat until eggs are cooked. Heat tortilla in microwave for 20 seconds. Lightly spread margarine on tortilla, then place eggs down the middle and roll up. Serves 1.

Optional: Add nonfat cheese and/or salsa. This will add a few more calories.

Calories: 126
Protein: 13 grams
Carbohydrates: 23 grams

Fat: 0.5 grams
Fiber: 2 grams
Sodium: 331 mg

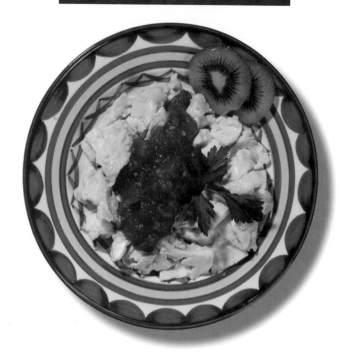

Scrambled Eggs with Salsa

6 egg whites + 1 yolk
Chunky salsa

Beat egg whites until bubbly. Spray a microwave bowl or saute' pan with non-stick spray. Cook in microwave for 45 seconds, stir. Cook another 45-60 seconds until eggs are cooked. Or, cook in small skillet over medium heat until eggs are cooked. Place on plate and top with salsa. Serves 1-2.

Calories: 157   *Fat: 5 grams*
Protein: 24 grams   *Fiber: 0 grams*
Carbohydrates: 2 grams   *Sodium: 310 mg*

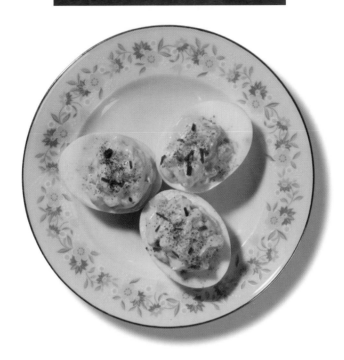

Deviled Eggs

4 hard-cooked eggs
1/4 cup nonfat mayonnaise
2 tablespoons dijon or yellow mustard
1/2 celery stalk, diced finely
Salt (optional)
Paprika

Slice eggs in half. Save two yolks and place in a bowl. Throw away the other yolks. Set aside 6 halved egg whites. Put other egg whites in bowl with yolks. Add all other ingredients and blend. Spoon yolk mixture into egg white halves. Sprinkle with paprika. Refrigerate. Serves 6 eggs.

Calories: 34   *Fat: 1.5 grams*
Protein: 5 grams   *Fiber: 0 grams*
Carbohydrates: 1 gram *Sodium: 130 mg*

SHAKES

Basic Protein Shake

Basic Protein Shake

4-6 ounces nonfat milk
5 tablespoons protein powder
(chocolate or vanilla)
Ice

Blend until smooth.

Calories: 178   *Fat: 0.3 grams*
Protein: 26 grams   *Fiber: 1 gram*
Carbohydrates: 13 grams *Sodium: 154 mg*

Basic Protein Shake Deluxe

12-16 ounces nonfat milk
10 tablespoons protein powder
(chocolate or vanilla)
Ice

Blend until smooth.

Calories: 356   *Fat: 0.6 grams*
Protein: 52 grams   *Fiber: 2 grams*
Carbohydrates: 26 grams *Sodium: 300 mg*

Banana Cream & Deluxe

Banana Cream Shake

Follow Basic Protein Shake recipe and
use vanilla protein powder and add 1
small banana.

Calories: 271   *Fat: 2.8 grams*
Protein: 27 grams   *Fiber: 3 grams*
Carbohydrates: 37 grams *Sodium: 155 mg*

Banana Cream Shake Deluxe

Follow recipe for Basic Protein Shake
Deluxe and use vanilla protein powder and
add 1 small banana.

Calories: 449   *Fat: 1.1 grams*
Protein: 53 grams   *Fiber: 4.4 grams*
Carbohydrates: 49 grams *Sodium: 310 mg*

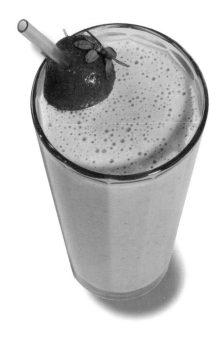

Strawberry & Deluxe

Strawberry Protein Shake

Follow Basic Protein Shake recipe and use vanilla protein powder and add 1 cup fresh or frozen strawberries.

Calories: 223　　*Fat: 0.9 grams*
Protein: 27 grams　　*Fiber: 4.5 grams*
Carbohydrates: 24 grams　　*Sodium: 156 mg*

Strawberry Protein Shake Deluxe

Follow recipe for Basic Protein Shake Deluxe and use vanilla protein powder and add 1-1/2 cups fresh or frozen strawberries.

Calories: 425　　*Fat: 1.5 grams*
Protein: 54 grams　　*Fiber: 7 grams*
Carbohydrates: 42 grams　　*Sodium: 310 mg*

Strawberry-Banana & Deluxe

Strawberry-Banana Shake

Follow Basic Protein Shake recipe and use vanilla protein powder. Add 1 cup strawberries and 1 small banana.

Calories: 317   *Fat: 1 gram*
Protein: 28 grams   *Fiber: 7 grams*
Carbohydrates: 47 grams *Sodium: 157 mg*

Strawberry-Banana Shake Deluxe

Follow recipe for Basic Protein Shake Deluxe and use vanilla protein powder. Add 1-1/2 cups fresh or frozen strawberries and 1 small banana.

Calories: 495   *Fat: 1.9 grams*
Protein: 54 grams   *Fiber: 8 grams*
Carbohydrates: 60 grams *Sodium: 311 mg*

French Vanilla & Deluxe

French Vanilla Protein Shake

Follow Basic Protein Shake recipe and use vanilla protein powder. Add 1 tablespoon Fat free French Vanilla coffee creamer.

Calories: 208   *Fat: 0.3 grams*
Protein: 26 grams   *Fiber: 1 gram*
Carbohydrates: 20 grams *Sodium 159 mg*

French Vanilla Protein Shake Deluxe

Follow recipe for Basic Protein Shake Deluxe and use vanilla protein powder. Add 2 tablespoons Fat-free French Vanilla coffee creamer.

Calories: 416   *Fat: 0.6 grams*
Protein: 52 grams   *Fiber: 2 grams*
Carbohydrates: 40 grams *Sodium: 310 mg*

Peanut butter & Deluxe

Peanut butter Protein Shake

Follow basic Protein Shake recipe and use vanilla or chocolate protein powder. Add 1 tablespoon peanut butter.

Calories: 273
Protein: 30 grams
bohydrates: 16 grams

Fat: 8.5 grams
Fiber: 2 grams Car-
Sodium: 229 mg

Peanut butter Protein Shake Deluxe

Follow recipe for Protein Shake Deluxe and use vanilla or chocolate protein powder. Add 2 tablespoons peanut butter.

Calories: 546
Protein: 60 grams
Carbohydrates: 32 grams

Fat: 17 grams
Fiber: 4 grams
Sodium: 458 mg

Peanut butter Strawberry & Deluxe

Peanut butter Strawberry Protein Shake

Follow Basic Protein Shake recipe and use vanilla or chocolate protein powder. Add 1 tablespoon peanut butter and 1 cup strawberries.

Calories: 319
Protein: 31 grams
Carbohydrates: 27 grams

Fat: 9 grams
Fiber: 5 grams
Sodium: 230 mg

Peanut butter Strawberry Protein Shake Deluxe

Follow recipe for Basic Protein Shake Deluxe and use vanilla or chocolate protein powder. Add 2 tablespoons peanut butter and 1-1/2 cup strawberries.

Calories: 592
Protein: 61 grams
Carbohydrates: 43 grams

Fat: 18 grams
Fiber: 7 grams
Sodium: 459 mg

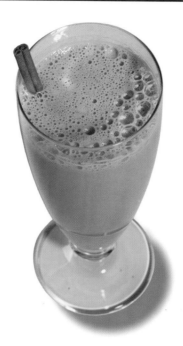

Cappuccino

3 ounces brewed coffee, cooled
3 ounces nonfat milk
5 tablespoons vanilla protein powder
Ice

Blend until smooth.

Calories: 145
Protein: 25 grams
Carbohydrates: 9 grams

Fat: 2 grams
Fiber: 1 gram
Sodium: 105 mg

Mocha & Deluxe

4 ounces cold brewed coffee
5 tablespoons chocolate protein powder
Ice

Blend until smooth.

Calories: 115
Protein: 20 grams
Carbohydrates: 4 grams

Fat: 2 grams
Fiber: 1 gram
Sodium: 60 mg

For Deluxe Mocha Shake:

Double the ingredients. Nutrition information will be double as well.

CHICKEN, TURKEY, FISH & BEEF

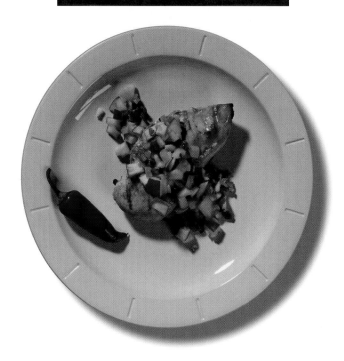

Washington Apple Salsa Chicken *by Sandi Anderson*

Salsa:

2 cups apple (Gala or Fuji) chopped
3/4 cup Anaheim Chili Peppers seeded
    and chopped
1/2 cup onion chopped
1/4 cup lime juice
2 tablespoons cilantro chopped

Mix and let stand at least 30 minutes.

Chicken:

2-1/2 pounds boneless skinless
    chicken breast
1/4 cup white wine
1/4 cup apple juice
1/2 teaspoon lime zest

Mix and marinate at least 20 minutes.

After chicken marinates, bake in oven at 350 for 45 minutes or grill on barbeque on low heat for 16-20 minutes, turning after 8 minutes. Serve salsa over cooked chicken. Serves 6.

Calories: 365   *Fat: 6 grams*
Protein: 58 grams   *Fiber: 0*
Carbohydrates: 10 grams   *Sodium: 144 mg*

BBQ Chicken Breast

<u>Quick and Large Volume</u>

2 pounds boneless, skinless chicken breast
8 tablespoons barbecue
   (hickory or original) sauce

Heat barbecue grill on high for 5 minutes. Reduce heat to low and spray grill with non-stick cooking spray. Place chicken breast on grill and cook for 8 minutes. Turn chicken over, and coat the cooked side of chicken with 1 tablespoon barbecue sauce. Cook chicken for another 8 minutes. Serves 8-4 ounce portions.

Calories: 146
Protein: 26 grams
Carbohydrates: 1 gram

Fat: 3 grams
Fiber: 0 grams
Sodium: 324 mg

Oven-fried Chicken

<u>Quick and Large Volume</u>

4 pounds boneless, skinless chicken breast
2 cups cornflakes crushed
1 tablespoon garlic powder
1 teaspoon seasoning salt
1 teaspoon paprika
2 cups skim milk

Preheat oven to 400 degrees. Mix dry ingredients in a quart size plastic bag. Dip chicken in milk and then place in bag and shake until chicken is coated. Place on a baking pan lined with foil. Cook chicken for 20-25 minutes. Serves 20-3 ounce portions.

Calories: 161
Protein: 28 grams
Carbohydrates: 3 grams

Fat: 3 grams
Fiber: 0 grams
Sodium: 408 mg

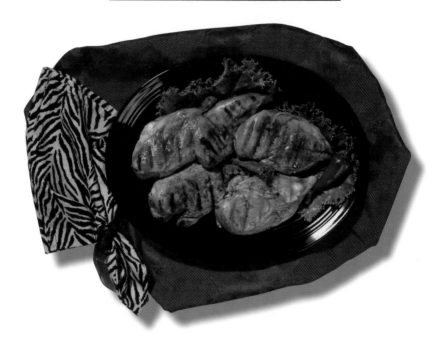

Sizzlin' Grilled Chicken Breast

Large Volume

2 pounds boneless, skinless chicken breast
Sizzlin' Grilling Marinade
   (see recipe, page 144)

Marinate chicken breast for at least 2 hours.
Prepare grill; spray with nonstick cooking
spray and reduce to low heat. Cook
chicken breast for 8-10 minutes on each
side until done. Serves 8-4 ounce portions.

Calories: 143
Protein: 26 gram
Carbohydrates: 1 gram

Fat: 3 grams
Fiber: 0 grams
Sodium: 260 mg

Baked Soy Sauce Chicken

Large Volume Recipe

5 pounds skinless, boneless chicken breast
1/2 cup reduced-sodium soy sauce
2 tablespoons garlic powder
water

Preheat oven to 350 degrees. Place chicken
in glass baking dish. Pour soy sauce over
chicken. Sprinkle with garlic. Add enough
water to fill dish with one inch of liquid.
Cover with foil and bake for 1 hour.
Makes 12-6 ounce servings.

Calories: 284
Protein: 53 grams
Carbohydrates: 0 grams

Fat: 6 grams
Fiber: 0 grams
Sodium: 300 mg

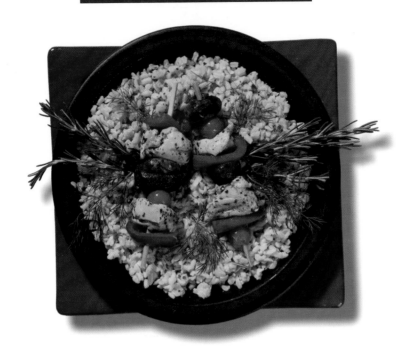

Chicken Brochettes *by Rosalie McPherson*

24 button mushrooms
  (2-8 ounce packages)
1-1/2 tablespoons Herbs de Province
  or Italian seasoning
2-1/2 tablespoons lime juice
1-1/2 tablespoons honey
1 teaspoon salt
1/2 teaspoon black pepper
1 pound skinless, boneless chicken breast
12-8 inch skewers
Cooking spray

Cut chicken breast into 24 pieces. Remove stems from mushrooms. Cook Herbs de Province in a small skillet with nonstick cooking spray over medium-low heat for 1 minute. Remove from heat and let cool. Stir in lime juice, honey, salt, and pepper. Place mushrooms and half of herb mixture in a large zip-lock plastic bag. Place chicken and remaining herb mixture in another plastic bag. Seal bags and marinate in the refrigerator for 1 hour, turning bags occasionally. Remove chicken and mushrooms from the bags and discard marinade. Preheat and prepare grill. Thread 4 mushrooms onto each of 6 skewers. Thread 4 chicken pieces onto each of the other 6 skewers. Place chicken brochettes on grill and cook for 5 minutes or until done over medium-low heat. Serves 6 (one of each skewer).

Calories: 160   *Fat: 1 gram*
Protein: 25 grams   *Fiber: 3 grams*
Carbohydrates: 8 grams *Sodium: 233 mg*

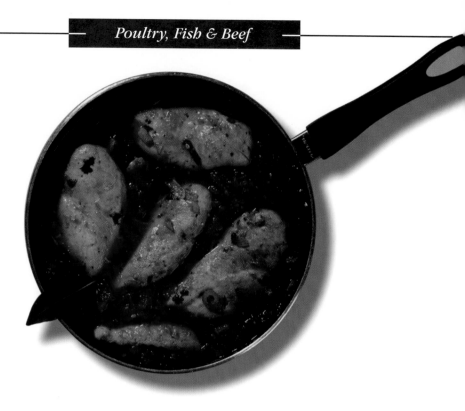

Bistro Chicken *by Jan Lutz*

6 boneless, skinless chicken breast halves
1 cup chopped onion
2 garlic cloves
1/2 cup chopped celery
1/4 cup chopped fresh basil
1/4 cup chopped fresh parsley
1/4 cup red wine vinegar
1/8 cup sliced olives
1/8 cup capers
2 teaspoons sugar
Dash of ground red pepper
1 bay leaf
1-14.5 ounce can Italian style tomatoes, diced

Spray a large skillet with nonstick cooking spray and place over medium-high heat. Add chicken, and sauté on each side until lightly browned. Remove from pan. Spray pan again. Add onion and garlic and saute' until translucent. Add celery and saute' for 5 minutes. Add basil, parsley, vinegar, olives, capers, sugar, red pepper, bay leaf and tomatoes. Return chicken to pan; bring to a boil. Cover, reduce heat, and simmer 20 minutes. Serve over pasta or rice. Serves 6 (1 chicken breast and 1/2 cup sauce).

Calories: 208   *Fat: 3.6 grams*
Protein: 29 grams   *Fiber: 2 grams*
Carbohydrates: 14 grams   *Sodium: 490 mg*

Apple-Turkey Kabobs

1 cup apple juice
2 tablespoons Worcestershire sauce
1/2 teaspoon lemon pepper
1 tablespoon garlic powder
1.5 pounds boneless, skinless turkey
    breast (1 inch cubes)
2 medium apples cut into wedges
1 large green pepper
18 mushrooms
Apple Barbeque Sauce
    (see recipe page 144)

Combine apple juice, Worcestershire sauce, lemon pepper, and garlic powder in large resealable plastic bag; add chicken turkey breast. Seal bag; turn to coat. Marinate in refrigerator for 2 hours. Heat barbeque grill. Prepare Apple Barbeque sauce; set aside. Remove meat from marinade an alternately thread meat, apple, and vegetables onto skewers. Spray grill with nonstick spray. Place kabobs on grill. Grill 10-12 minutes turning after 6 minutes, occasionally brushing with Apple Barbeque sauce. Serves 6.

Calories: 173
Protein: 29 grams
Carbohydrates: 11 grams

Fat: 1 gram
Fiber: 2 grams
Sodium: 142 mg

Turkey Meatloaf

<u>Large Volume</u>

2 pounds ground turkey breast
4 egg whites
2 tablespoons garlic powder
3 slices nonfat cheese
1/2 cup barbecue sauce

Preheat oven to 350 degrees. Mix turkey breast, garlic and egg whites together and place in rectangular baking dish forming a loaf. Cover with foil and bake for 45 minutes. Uncover and place slices of cheese on top of loaf, then pour barbecue sauce over the top. Leave uncovered and bake for another 15 minutes. Serves 8.

Calories: 185
Protein: 36 grams
Carbohydrates: 7 grams

Fat: 2 grams
Fiber: 0.6 grams
Sodium: 312 mg

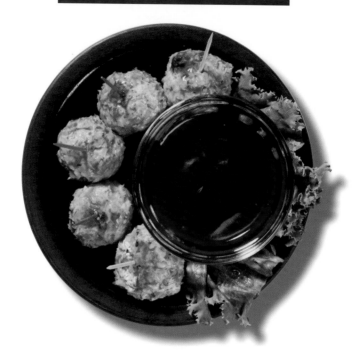

Turkey Meatballs *by Rosalie McPherson*

<u>Quick and Large Volume</u>

2.5 pounds ground turkey breast
1/4 cups old fashioned oatmeal (dry)
1-1/2 cups brown rice (cooked)
3 jumbo egg whites
1/4 teaspoon salt
1-1/2 teaspoon sage
1/4 teaspoon thyme
1-1/2 teaspoon onion powder
1/4 teaspoon black pepper

Mix all ingredients. Form 6 meatballs for every one cup of mixture. Bake at 425 degrees on a foil-lined baking sheet, sprayed with nonstick cooking spray for 4-6 minutes, then turn over and cook another 4-6 minutes. One meatball:

Calories: 91
Protein: 6 grams
Carbohydrates: 14 grams

Fat: 0.5 grams
Fiber: 1 gram
Sodium: 172 mg

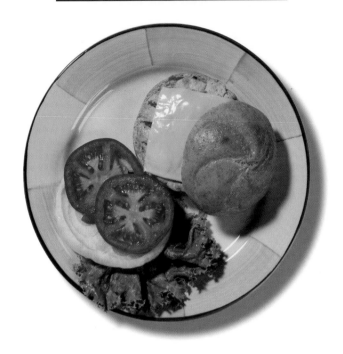

Turkey Salsa Burgers

Quick and Large Volume

2.5 pounds ground turkey breast
1 cup thick and chunky salsa
3 tablespoons powdered garlic

Heat barbeque grill. Turn to low. Mix all ingredients in large bowl. Make eight patties. Spray grill with cooking spray. Cook turkey for 7-9 minutes on each side. Do not overcook turkey or it will be very dry. Makes 8-3 ounce servings.

Calories: 133
Protein: 27 grams
Carbohydrates: 3 grams

Fat: 1.5 grams
Fiber: 0 grams
Sodium: 230 mg

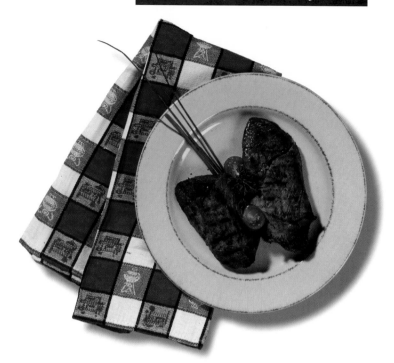

Grilled Pepper Steak

<u>Quick</u>

2 pounds lean top sirloin steaks
1/2 cup chicken broth
1/4 cup chopped fresh parsley
1/4 cup minced onion
2 tablespoons Worcestershire sauce
1 teaspoon freshly ground pepper
1/2 teaspoon dry mustard

Combine broth, parsley, onion and Worcestershire sauce and mustard in a sauce pan. Heat, stirring continually for 3 minutes. Heat grill and place steaks on low heat. Brush with pepper mixture frequently. Depending on thickness of steaks, cook about 6-8 minutes on each side for a medium steak. Serves 8.

Calories: 175   *Fat: 7 grams*
Protein: 26 grams   *Fiber: 0*
Carbohydrates: 0   *Sodium: 89 mg*

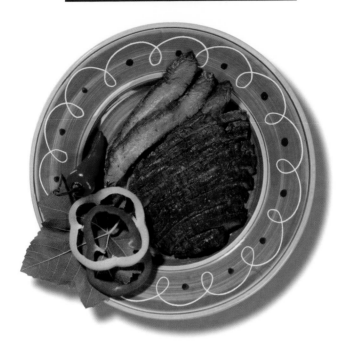

Marinated Flank Steak *by Jan Lutz*

1 pound lean flank steak
1/3 cup dry red wine
1/4 cup chopped sweet onion
2 teaspoons reduced-sodium soy sauce
2 garlic cloves, minced
1/4 teaspoon salt
1/4 teaspoon pepper
Cooking spray

Combine wine, onion, soy sauce, garlic, salt and pepper in a large zip-lock bag. Add steak to bag. Seal and marinate for at least 30 minutes, turning occasionally. Prepare grill. Place steak on grill rack coated with cooking spray. Grill 5 minutes on each side until desired degree of doneness. Cut steak diagonally across the grain in thin slices. Serves 4.

Calories: 311
Protein: 36 grams
Carbohydrates: 1 gram

Fat: 14 grams
Fiber: 0 grams
Sodium: 442 mg

Fish with Cucumber Relish

<u>Quick</u>

1 can (11 ounces) mandarin oranges, drained
1 small cucumber, peeled, finely chopped
1/3 cup rice vinegar
1 green onion, minced
1 tablespoon dill
1 pound orange roughy

Reserve 8 sections of mandarin oranges fo garnish; coarsely chop remaining sections and combine with cucumber, vinegar, onion and dill. Spray broiler pan with cooking spray; place fish on pan. Spoon 1 tablespoon cucumber mixture over each fillet. Broil for 8-10 minutes or until fish is cooked. To serve, top with remaining relish mix and garnish will orange sections and dill sprigs. Serves 4.

Calories: 146   *Fat: 1 gram*
Protein: 21 grams   *Fiber: 1 gram*
Carbohydrates: 13 grams *Sodium: 67 mg*

Microwave Cod Fillets

<u>Quick</u>

1 pound cod or orange roughy
3/4 cup nonfat sour cream
1/4 cup nonfat mayonnaise
3 tablespoons skim milk
1 tablespoon dijon mustard
1-1/2 teaspoon dill

Cut fish into 4 pieces; place in a microwave-safe dish. Cover and microwave on high for 2-4 minutes. Drain and combine the sour cream, mayonnaise, milk, mustard and dill. Drizzle 1/2 cup over fish and microwave uncovered for 3-4 minutes or until fish flakes easily with a fork. Serves 4.

Calories: 128   *Fat: 1.3 grams*
Protein: 22 grams   *Fiber: 0*
Carbohydrates: 6 grams *Sodium: 164 mg*

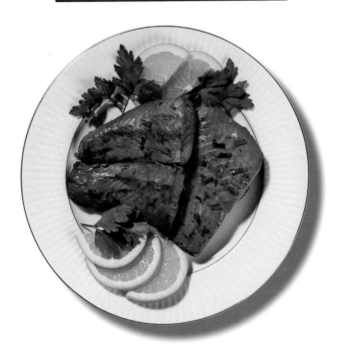

Grilled Salmon

1 pound fresh salmon
1/2 reduced-sodium soysauce
1 tablespoon brown sugar
1/4 cup lemon juice
1 teaspoon grated lemon peel

Mix all ingredients in a large plastic storage bag. Divide salmon into 4 pieces.

Place salmon in bag and marinate for 1 hour. Broil fish for 3-4 minutes on each side until fish flakes easily with fork.
Makes 4-4 ounce servings.

Calories: 342   *Fat: 19 grams*
Protein: 36 grams   *Fiber: 0*
Carbohydrates: 8 grams *Sodium: 1061 mg*

Foil-baked Salmon

Quick

1 pound salmon
1/2 lemon, sliced thin
2 tablespoons lemon pepper

Place fish on a large piece of foil. Sprinkle lemon pepper over fish and lay lemon

wedges on top of fish. Wrap up in foil and bake in preheated oven of 350 degrees. Bake for 20 minutes or until fish flakes with a fork. Serves 4.

Calories: 326   *Fat: 18 grams*
Protein: 34 grams   *Fiber: 0*
Carbohydrates: 5 grams *Sodium: 101 mg*

Sizzlin' Grilling Marinade

1 cup Worcestershire sauce
1 cup vinegar (red wine or rice)
1/2 cup teriyaki or gourmet sauce
1 tablespoon dijon mustard
1 tablespoon garlic powder

Mix all ingredients. Marinate steak, chicken or turkey breasts for at least 2 hours. Left over marinade can be froze and reused. Cook meat on low-heat grill to desired doneness. Serves 32 or 1 teaspoon servings.

Calories: 9   *Fat: 0 grams*
Protein: 0 grams   *Fiber: 0 grams*
Carbohydrates: 2 gramss   *Sodium: 205 mg*

Spicy Marinade

1/4 cup reduced-sodium soy sauce
1/4 cup orange juice
2 teaspoons sugar substitute
2 cloves of garlic
1 teaspoon rum extract
1/4 teaspoon ground ginger
1 teaspoon hot pepper sauce

Mix all ingredients in a resealable plastic bag. Put uncooked chicken or turkey breast in marinade for 2 hours.

Calories: 21   *Fat: 0 grams*
Protein: 0 grams   *Fiber: 0 grams*
Carbohydrates: 5 grams   *Sodium: 301 mg*

Apple Barbeque Sauce

1/2 cup chopped onion
1/2 cup apple juice
1 cup chili sauce
1/2 cup unsweetened applesauce
2 teaspoons sugar substitute
1 tablespoon Worcestershire sauce
1 teaspoon dry mustard
5 drops hot pepper sauce

Combine onion and apple juice in 1 quart saucepan. Simmer for 2 minutes. Stir in chili sauce, applesauce, sugar, Worcestershire sauce, mustard and pepper sauce. Simmer 10 minutes. Makes 2 cups.

2 tablespoons of sauce:

Calories: 31   *Fat: 0 grams*
Protein: 0 grams   *Fiber: 0 grams*
Carbohydrates: 8 grams   *Sodium: 211 mg*

MAIN ENTREES

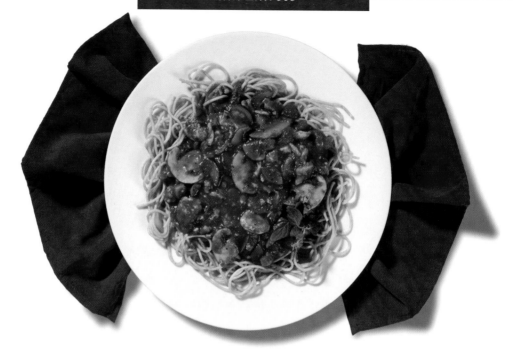

Spaghetti Sauce

1 pound ground turkey breast
1 small onion
12 ounces sliced mushrooms
1 green pepper, diced
2 small zucchinis diced
1-15 ounce Italian stewed tomatoes
3-8 ounce tomato sauce
1 tablespoon garlic powder
2-6 ounce tomato paste
1 teaspoon each of oregano, basil and salt
  (optional)

In an extra large skillet, spray with nonstick spray. Add meat and onion. Brown meat. Dice and slice vegetables and add with all other ingredients. Simmer until vegetables are tender (1-2 hours). Serves 12-1 cup servings.

Calories: 101   *Fat: 0.6 grams*
Protein: 14 grams   *Fiber: 3 grams*
Carbohydrates: 11 grams *Sodium: 467mg*

Vegetarian Spaghetti Sauce

Eliminate meat. This will decrease the calories to 61; protein 6 grams and fat 0 grams.

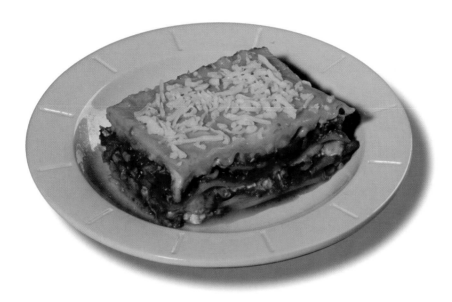

Turkey Lasagna

1 pound ground turkey breast
1 tablespoon garlic powder
12 ounces mushrooms, sliced
1 green pepper
1-15 ounce diced stewed tomatoes,
    drained
2-8 ounce tomato sauce
2-6 ounce tomato paste
1 teaspoon each of oregano, basil and
    salt (optional)
1-16 ounce nonfat cottage cheese
4 egg whites
8 ounces nonfat shredded mozarella
8 ounces nonfat shredded cheddar cheese
10 wide lasagna noodles

In large skillet, brown meat with garlic powder. Add mushrooms, pepper, tomatoes, sauce, paste, and spices. This is your meat sauce. Cook your noodles until tender. Mix cottage cheese and egg whites. In 13x9 baking dish, lay three noodles on the bottom. Spoon on half of the meat sauce over noodles Spread half of the cottage cheese mixture over sauce. Sprinkle 1/3 of each of the shredded cheeses over the meat/cottage cheese. Make another layer of the noodles, then meat sauce, cottage cheese mix and cheeses. For the top, lay the last three noodles. Sprinkle with the remaining 1/3 of each of the shredded cheeses. Cover with foil and bake at 350 degrees for 1 hour. Serves 12.

Calories: 219   *Fat: 1.5 grams*
Protein: 28 grams   *Fiber: 2.6 grams*
Carbohydrates: 26 grams   *Sodium: 702 mg*

Vegetarian Lasagna

Eliminate the turkey. This will reduce the calories to 175; protein 17 grams; and fat 1 gram.

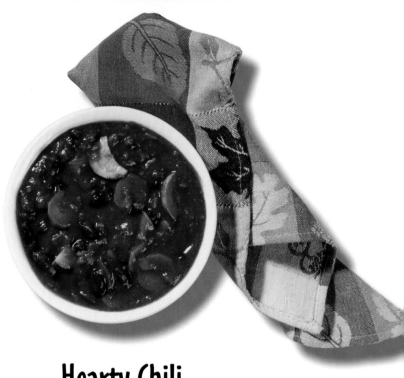

Hearty Chili

1 pound ground turkey breast
   or 4% lean ground beef
1 small onion
3 zucchini
1 green pepper
1 large carrot
1-15 ounce stewed tomatoes
3-15 ounce low sodium kidney beans
1-15 ounce black beans
3-15 ounce tomato sauce
2 teaspoons chili powder
1 tablespoon garlic powder
1 teaspoon salt (optional)
2-8 ounce tomato paste

In large stock or crock pot, brown meat. Slice and dice vegetables. Add vegetables and all other ingredients to meat. Simmer until vegetables are tender (1-3 hours). Makes 20-1 cup servings.

Calories: 197   *Fat: 1 gram*
Protein: 20 grams   *Fiber: 8 grams*
Carbohydrates: 28 grams   *Sodium: 814 mg*

Vegetarian Chili

Eliminate the meat. This will reduce the calories to 169; protein 14 grams; and fat 0.2 grams.

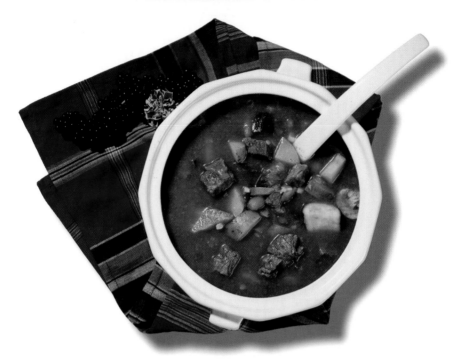

Beef Stew

2 pounds flank Steak
2-15 ounce tomato sauce
12 ounces mushrooms, sliced
16 ounces baby carrots
1 pound red potatos with skin
2 tablespoon garlic powder
4 zucchini, cut into 1" chuncks
1 teaspoon basil
1 teaspoon salt (optional)
12 cups water
12 chicken bouillon cubes

Cut up meat in 1 inch cubes. In large stock or crock pot, brown meat with onions. Add tomato sauce and boil for 30 minutes. Add all the other ingredients. Simmer for 1-3 hours until potatoes are tender. Serves 16.

Calories: 192   *Fat: 3 grams*
Protein: 19 grams   *Fiber: 2 grams*
Carbohydrates: 19 grams   *Sodium: 396 mg*

Oriental Chicken Noodle Soup

7 ounces whole wheat spaghetti noodles,
   dry
12.5 ounces chicken breast, canned
1 large carrot
1 celery Stalk
1 tablespoon reduced-sodium soy sauce
8 bouillon cubes
8 cups of water

Heat water and dissolve bouillon cubes. Add noodles, celery, carrot and soy sauce. Cook until tender. Add chicken and simmer on low for 15 minutes. Serves 8.

Calories: 171   *Fat: 2 grams*
Protein: 18 grams   *Fiber: 0*
Carbohydrates: 20 grams   *Sodium: 1001 mg*

Angel Hair Pasta with Chicken

12 ounces chicken breast, cubed
1 large carrot, sliced diagonally into
    1/4 inch pieces
10 ounce package of frozen broccoli
    florets
2 cloves garlic, minced
12 ounces angel hair pasta
2/3 cup chicken broth
1 teaspoon dried basil
1/4 cup grated parmesan cheese

Spray medium skillet with nonstick spray. Heat and add chicken breast. Cook, stirring until chicken is cooked through, about 5 minutes. Remove from skillet. Begin heating water for pasta. In skillet, add carrot and 3 tablespoons of chicken broth and cook for 4 minutes. Add garlic and broccoli to skillet and cook for another 2 minutes. Cook pasta according to directions. While pasta is cooking, add the rest of the chicken broth, basil and chicken in skillet. Simmer for 4 minutes. Drain pasta. Place in large serving bowl. Top with chicken mixture and then parmesan cheese. Serves 4.

Calories: 493   *Fat: 6.5 grams*
Protein: 44 grams   *Fiber: 2 grams*
Carbohydrates: 68 grams   *Sodium: 534 mg*

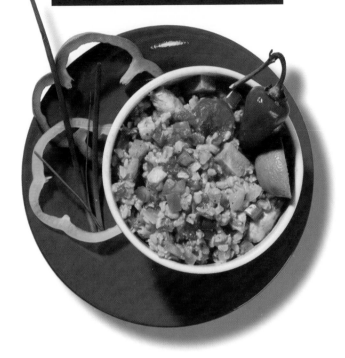

Chicken or Shrimp Jambalaya *by Jan Lutz*

1 medium onion
2 garlic cloves
1 pound chicken breast cut into 3/4 inch
    pieces or 1 pound of shrimp
1-14.5 ounce can whole plum tomatoes
1 tablespoon tomato paste
1 celery stalk, cut into 1/2 inch slices
1 small green pepper, seeded and
    chopped
1 whole scallion
1 bay leaf
1 teaspoon dried thyme
Pinch ground clove
1/4 teaspoon red pepper flakes
4 ounce of lean ham, cut into 1/2
    inch cubes
1 cup long-grain brown rice, cooked

In a 3 quart Dutch oven, saute the onion and garlic in nonstick cooking spray over medium-high heat, about 4 minutes. Add the chicken and cook, stirring until the pieces are white on all sides. Add the undrained tomatoes, and all the rest of the ingredients except for the rice and ham. Bring to a boil and simmer until the chicken is cooked and the sauce has thickened, about 20 minutes. Mix the ham and rice into the chicken mixture, heat and serve. Makes 6 servings.

Calories: 169   *Fat: 2 grams*
Protein: 23 grams   *Fiber: 2 grams*
Carbohydrates: 14 grams   *Sodium: 439 mg*

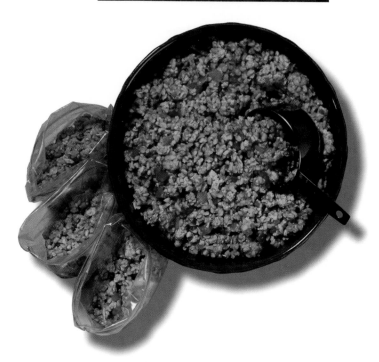

Turkey Rice Mix *by Blair McHaney*

Large Volume Recipe

3.35 pounds ground turkey breast
3 cups brown rice

Optional seasonings:
   Garlic, italian, taco, pepper, Mrs. Dash,
   salsa, or seasoned rice vinegar

Optional:
   3 cups of mixed vegetables
      (broccoli, green beans, stir-fry)
      or 3 cups chopped apples

Cook the rice. Cook the turkey breast with the seasoning. Mix in very large bowl. Use containers or quart size baggies for refrigeration or freezing. Decide how many bags you will need from the following breakdown. Fill each bag or container evenly until mixture is gone. Adding vegetables or apples will add a small amount of calories. This will also add extra fiber and variety. This recipe is also tasty without adding seasoning during the cooking, but rather after it's reheated. Use these prepared meals for between meal snacks or main entrees.

Divided:	Calories	Protein-grams	Fat-grams	Carbs-grams	Fiber	Sodium-mg
10 meals	387	39	2.6	47	3	137
12 meals	322	32	2.2	39.5	2.5	119
15 meals	258	26	1.75	31.5	2	106

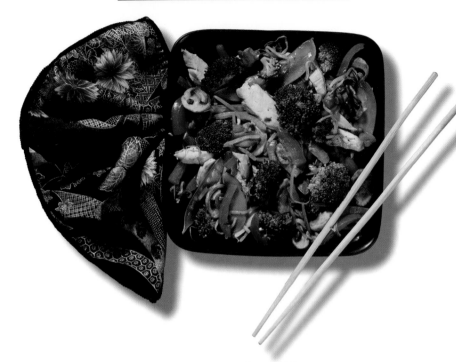

Chicken Stir-Fry

1 pound boneless, skinless chicken
  breast
4 cups broccoli flowerets
4 cups mushrooms, sliced
3 cups sugar snap peas
2 cups bean sprouts
1 green, or red pepper, seeded, sliced
1 small onion, chopped

Cut chicken into strips. Heat in wok or large skillet coated with nonstick spray. Brown chicken. Add onions and green peppers. Sauté on medium for 3 minutes. Add other ingredients, cover and cook until crisp tender, about 5-6 minutes. Serves 4.

Calories: 319   *Fat: 5 grams*
Protein: 43 grams   *Fiber: 12 grams*
Carbohydrates: 30 grams *Sodium: 212 mg*

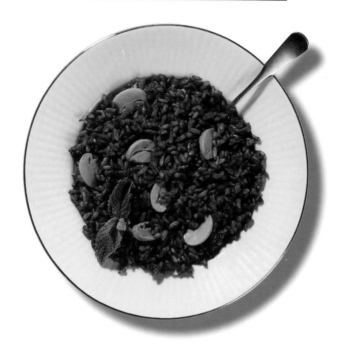

Tasty Brown Rice

Brown, basmati, wild, long grain rice
Bouillion cubes or fat-free chicken broth
Water

Prepare rice as directed on package. For each cup of water, use one bouillon cube or replace water by using only fat-free chicken broth. Cook as directed. 1 cup serving:

Calories: 235
Protein: 5 grams
Carbohydrates: 50 grams

Fat: 1 gram
Fiber: 3 grams
Sodium: 1126 mg

Chicken Apple Stir-fry *by Royce Tigner*

4 ounces dried mushrooms, shiitake
   or wood ear
12 ounces skinless, boneless chicken
   breast
3/4 cup water
3 tablespoons frozen orange juice
   concentrate, thawed
2 tablespoons low-sodium soy sauce
2 teaspoons cornstarch
1/4 teaspoon ground ginger
1/4 teaspoon ground cinnamon
1/4 teaspoon ground red pepper
3 tablespoons sliced or slivered almonds
2 medium green peppers, cut into
   2" strips
2 medium apples, thinly sliced

In small bowl, add warm water to mushrooms and soak for 30 minutes. Rinse and squeeze mushrooms to drain thoroughly. Discard stems. Thinly slice mushrooms and set aside. Rinse chicken and pat dry. Cut into 1 inch pieces. Set aside. In a small bowl, stir together cold water, juice concentrate, soy sauce, cornstarch, ginger, cinnamon, and red pepper. Set aside. Preheat skillet or wok over medium-high heat. Spray with nonstick cooking spray and add almonds; stir-fry for 2-3 minutes or until golden. Remove almonds from skillet. Spray skillet with nonstick cooking spray. Add mushrooms, peppers and apples; stir-fry for 1-2 minutes or until peppers and apples are crisp-tender. Remove apple mixture from skillet. Add chicken to skillet and stir-fry for 3-4 minutes or until browned. Push chicken from center of skillet. Stir sauce and add to the center of skillet. Cook and stir until thickened and bubbly. Return apple mixture to the wok. Stir all ingredients together to coat with sauce. Cook and stir 1-2 minutes or until heated thoroughly. Stir in toasted almonds. Serves 4.

Calories: 220   *Fat: 5 grams*
Protein: 24 grams   *Fiber: 4.5 grams*
Carbohydrates: 22 grams *Sodium: 180 mg*

Serve over 1/2 cup brown rice:
Calories: 337   *Fat: 5 grams*
Protein: 26 grams   *Fiber: 6 grams*
Carbohydrates: 47 grams *Sodium: 195 mg*

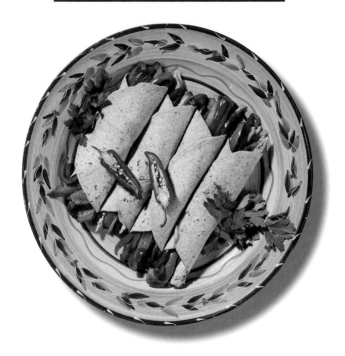

Fajita's — Beef or Chicken

1 pound top-sirloin or chicken breast
   strips cooked
1 small onion, cut in strips
1 green pepper, cut in strips
1 red pepper, cut in strips
1 tablespoon chili powder
1 tablespoon garlic powder
Chicken broth
5 whole wheat tortillas

Sauté onions and peppers in broth until tender. In same pan, add meat to one side of the pan. Add chili and garlic powder and simmer all for 20 minutes on low heat. Heat tortillas in microwave. Makes 5 tortillas.

Using 3 ounces of chicken breast:

Calories: 236	*Fat: 3.5 grams*
Protein: 30 grams	*Fiber: 2.6 grams*
Carbohydrates: 26 grams	*Sodium: 494 mg*

Using 3 ounce of beef:

Calories: 260	*Fat: 6 grams*
Protein: 29 grams	*Fiber: 2.6 grams*
Carbohydrates: 26 grams	*Sodium: 495 mg*

Whole Wheat Tortilla Tacos

1 pound ground turkey breast or 4% lean
    ground beef
5 whole wheat tortillas (35 grams)
1 packet taco seasoning mix
5 ounces nonfat shredded cheddar cheese
Lettuce and salsa

Cook meat until browned. Follow the directions on using the seasoning packet. Warm tortillas in microwave for 10-15 seconds. Use 3 ounces of meat and 1 ounce of cheese on each tortilla. Add desired amount of lettuce and salsa. Serves 5.

Using Beef:
Calories: 278	*Fat: 7 grams*
Protein: 35 grams	*Fiber: 2 grams*
Carbohydrates: 22 grams	*Sodium: 969 mg*

Using turkey breast:
Calories: 207	*Fat: 2 grams*
Protein: 32 grams	*Fiber: 2 grams*
Carbohydrates: 23 grams	*Sodium: 981 mg*

Corn Tortilla Tacos

1 pound ground turkey breast of 4% lean
    ground beef
10 corn tortilla (4")
1 packet taco seasoning mix
5 ounces nonfat shredded cheddar cheese
Lettuce and salsa

Cook meat until browned. Follow the directions on using the seasoning packet. Warm corn tortillas in microwave for 10-15 seconds. Use 1-1/2 ounce of meat and 1/2 ounce of cheese on each tortilla. Add desired amount of lettuce and salsa. Serving size is 2 tortillas.

Using Beef:
Calories: 240	*Fat: 7 grams*
Protein: 33 grams	*Fiber: 1 gram*
Carbohydrates: 10 grams	*Sodium: 812 mg*

Using turkey breast:
Calories: 170	*Fat: 2 grams*
Protein: 30 grams	*Fiber: 1 gram*
Carbohydrates: 10 grams	*Sodium: 825 mg*

Bean Burrito

2 cups nonfat refried beans
4 whole wheat tortillas
4 ounces of nonfat shredded
   cheddar cheese
Salsa

Place 1/2 cup beans, 1 ounce of cheese, and 2 tablespoons salsa on each tortilla. Roll up and place all tortillas in microwave baking dish. Heat for 2-3 minutes until cheese melts. Serves 5.

Calories: 213   *Fat: 1 gram*
Protein: 15 grams   *Fiber: 6.5 grams*
Carbohydrates: 42 grams   *Sodium: 644 mg*

Beef Burrito

1 pound 4% ground beef
5 whole wheat tortillas
5 ounces nonfat shredded cheddar cheese
Salsa and desired spices (garlic powder)

Brown meat and drain. Heat tortillas in microwave for 10-15 seconds. Place 3 ounces of meat, 1 ounce of cheese and desired amount of salsa on tortilla and roll up. Heat in microwave for 25 seconds. Serves 5.

Calories: 277   *Fat: 7 grams*
Protein: 35 grams   *Fiber: 2 grams*
Carbohydrates: 22 grams   *Sodium: 487 mg*

Beef & Bean Burrito

1 pound 4% ground beef
1-1/4 cup nonfat refried beans
5 whole wheat tortillas
5 ounces nonfat shredded cheddar cheese
Salsa and desired spices (garlic powder)

Brown meat and spices and drain. Heat tortillas in microwave for 10-15 seconds. Place 3 ounce of meat, 1 ounce of cheese, 1/4 cup beans, and desired amount of salsa on tortilla and roll up. Heat all tortillas in microwave for 2-3 minutes. Serves 5.

Calories: 331   *Fat: 7 grams*
Protein: 38 grams   *Fiber: 4 grams*
Carbohydrates: 32 grams   *Sodium: 587 mg*

"No Stick 'Um" Apple Pizza *by Mary Ellen Kerby*

Crust: Mix dry ingredients, then add liquids. Roll out crust and place on a 12 inch pizza pan.

1-1/2 cups stone ground whole wheat flour

1 tablespoon sugar substitute

1 package yeast (dissolve in 1/2 cup 110 degree F water)

1/2 teaspoon salt

1 tablespoon unsweetened applesauce

1 tablespoon olive oil

1/2 teaspoon vanilla extract

Topping:

3/4 tablespoon "light" margarine

2 cups shredded low-fat mozzarella or cheddar cheese

4 medium apples, peeled and thinly sliced

Cinnamon and sugar substitute

Brush dough with margarine. Sprinkle cinnamon and sugar substitute evenly over dough. Spread cheese over dough, and place apple slices on top of cheese. Sprinkle again with cinnamon and sugar substitute. Bake at 375 degrees for 25 minutes. Serves 8-10.

Calories: 181	*Fat: 3 grams*
Protein: 9.6 grams	*Fiber: 4.6 grams*
Carbohydrates: 31 grams	*Sodium: 596 mg*

Sweet Tater Surprise *by Nancy Van Hoven*

1/3 cup water

1/3 cup old fashioned oatmeal, uncooked

3 tablespoons vanilla protein powder

1 medium sweet potato, cooked

Remove skin on cooked sweet potato and mash. Mix with water, oatmeal and protein powder. Serves 8-10.

Calories: 238	*Fat: 0.8 grams*
Protein: 11 grams	*Fiber: 7 grams*
Carbohydrates: 48 grams	*Sodium: 29 mg*

SALADS & VEGETABLES

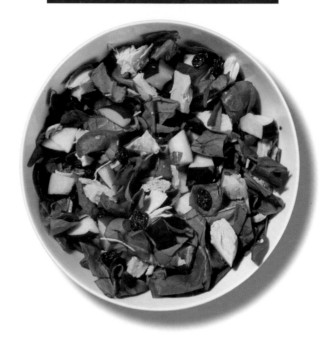

Waldorf Salad

3 ounces cooked chicken breast
2 cup spinach, chopped
1 medium apple, chopped
1/2 tablespoon walnuts
1 teaspoon raisins
2 tablespoons nonfat salad dressing
   (Honey mustard or Catalina)

Dice chicken breast. Toss all ingredients together and add salad dressing.
1 serving.

Calories: 313   *Fat: 6 grams*
Protein: 29 grams   *Fiber: 7 grams*
Carbohydrates: 38 grams   *Sodium: 398 mg*

Grilled Chicken Caesar

3 ounces chicken breast, grilled
2 cups romaine lettuce, chopped
1 tablespoon shredded parmesan
2 tablespoons nonfat caesar salad dressing

Cut chicken breast into strips. Mix all ingredients in a bowl and serve. 1 serving.

Calories: 192   *Fat: 5 grams*
Protein: 30 grams   *Fiber: 2 grams*
Carbohydrates: 6 grams   *Sodium: 345 mg*

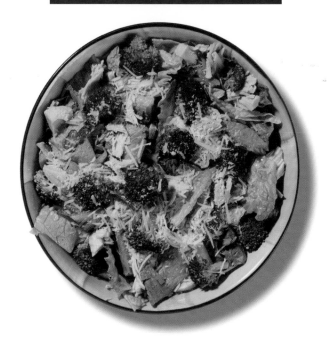

Chicken-Broccoli Salad

3 ounces chicken breast, canned
1 cup broccoli, chopped
2 cups romaine lettuce, chopped
1/2 tablespoon shredded parmesan
2 tablespoons nonfat salad dressing

Cut chicken into 1" cubes. Toss with lettuce, broccoli and salad dressing. Sprinkle parmesan over the top. 1 serving.

Calories: 221   *Fat: 4 grams*
Protein: 31 grams   *Fiber: 5 grams*
Carbohydrates: 16 grams *Sodium: 602 mg*

Chicken-Apple Lettuce Salad

3-1/2 cups diced red apples
2 tablespoons lemon juice
2 cups grapes
1 celery stalk, diced
1 large carrot, shredded
3 cups romaine lettuce, chopped
12 ounces canned chicken breast
1/3 cup walnut pieces
1/2 cup nonfat mayonnaise
2 tablespoons nonfat sour cream

Mix apples with lemon juice. In separate bowl, mix mayonnaise and sour cream. Add other ingredients to the apples. Toss, then add the mayonnaise mixture and mix well. Serves 8.

Calories: 200   *Fat: 4 grams*
Protein: 11 grams   *Fiber: 4 grams*
Carbohydrates: 33 grams *Sodium: 935 mg*

Smoked Turkey Apple Salad *by Gloria and Stanley Arbogast*

Dressing-Mix together:

1 tablespoon olive oil
1 tablespoon dijon mustard
2 tablespoons apple cider vinegar
1 teaspoon lemon pepper

Salad- Toss together:

8 cups romaine lettuce, chopped
1 carrot, julienne
10 cherry tomatoes, halved
8 ounces smoked turkey breast, julienne
4 unpeeled apples, diced
2 tablespoons chopped walnuts, toasted

Arrange lettuce on a platter or plates. Top with salad ingredients except walnuts, then drizzle salad dressing on top and finish with a sprinkle of walnuts over the salad.
Serves 4.

Calories: 209   *Fat: 7 grams*
Protein: 15 grams   *Fiber: 4.5 grams*
Carbohydrates: 24 grams *Sodium: 817 mg*

Oriental Salmon Salad

6 ounces salmon
1-1/2 cups red cabbage, shredded
8 cups chinese cabbage, shredded
2 cups carrots, shredded
1 cup sliced green onions
1 can mandarine oranges (10 ounces)
1/4 cup slivered almonds
5 ounces rice noodles
1 bottle nonfat oriental dressing

Mix all ingredients except the salmon and noodles. Gently mix in salmon and top with rice noodles. Makes 6-2 cup servings.

Calories: 363   *Fat: 5.8 grams*
Protein: 12 grams   *Fiber: 4 grams*
Carbohydrates: 65 grams *Sodium: 723 mg*

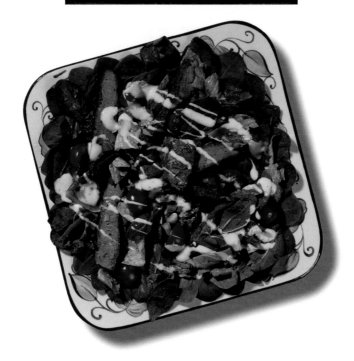

Steak Salad

3 ounces top sirloin steak grilled
1/2 green pepper, seeded, cut in strips
1/2 small onion, cut in strips
2 cups romaine lettuce
1 cup spinach
2 tablespoons nonfat ranch dressing

Sauté pepper and onion in pan with non-stick spray until crisp tender. Cut steak into strips and add to pan. Heat for 2 minutes. Chop lettuce and spinach. Mix in dressing until evenly distributed. Add meat mixture and serve. 1 serving.

Calories: 237   *Fat: 6 grams*
Protein: 29 grams   *Fiber: 5 grams*
Carbohydrates: 17 grams *Sodium: 362 mg*

Tuna Mixed Green Salad

6 ounces tuna in water, drained
2 cups romaine lettuce
1 cup spinach
1 small tomato
2 tablespoons nonfat italian dressing

Chop lettuce, spinach and tomato. Toss in tuna and mix. Add dressing. Serves 1.

Calories: 268   *Fat: 2 grams*
Protein: 46 grams   *Fiber: 3 grams*
Carbohydrates: 14 grams *Sodium: 961 mg*

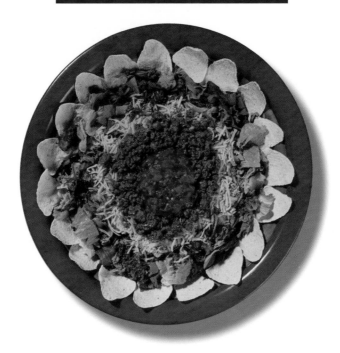

Taco Salad

1 pound 4% lean ground beef
 or ground turkey breast
1 packet taco seasoning mix
8 cups mixed green lettuce
4 ounces nonfat cheddar cheese
2 cups salsa

Cook meat until brown. Prepare and add seasoning as directed on package to meat. Chop lettuce and place in a bowl. Add 1/4 of meat, 1 ounce of cheese and 1/2 cup salsa over lettuce. Serves 4.

Calories: 236   *Fat: 5 grams*
Protein: 30 grams   *Fiber: 7 grams*
Carbohydrates: 19 grams   *Sodium: 1137 mg*

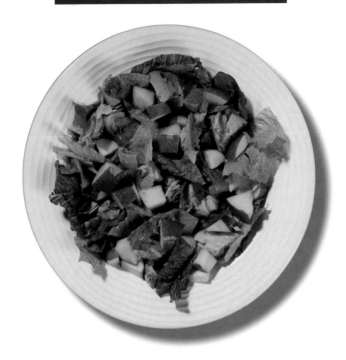

Grilled Salmon Salad

3 ounces grilled salmon
2 cups romaine lettuce
1 cup chopped zucchini
1 medium apple
2 tablespoon seasoned rice vinegar

Chop lettuce and mix all the ingredients.
1 serving.

Calories: 288   *Fat: 7 grams*
Protein: 22 grams   *Fiber: 11 grams*
Carbohydrates: 27 grams   *Sodium: 64 mg*

Salmon Caesar

3 ounces salmon, canned or grilled
2 cups romaine lettuce chopped
1 tablespoon shredded parmesan
2 tablespoons nonfat caesar salad dressing

Chunk salmon. Mix all ingredients
in a bowl and serve. 1 serving.

Calories: 174   *Fat: 7.5 grams*
Protein: 21 grams   *Fiber: 2 grams*
Carbohydrates: 6 grams   *Sodium: 438 mg*

Fresh Vegetable Stir-Fry

1 tablespoon cornstarch
1/2 teaspoon salt
1 cup chicken broth
1/4 pound green beans,
   cut into 1 1/2 inch pieces
3 small onions
1 large clove garlic, minced
1 medium zucchini
1 large green or red pepper,
   cut into thin strips
1/2 cup thinly sliced carrots
1 medium tomato, cut into wedges
1/4 cup minced fresh basil
1 teaspoon lemon juice (optional)

In small bowl, stir cornstarch, salt and broth until smooth; set aside. Spray large skillet with nonstick cooking spray and heat on medium-high heat. Add beans, onions and garlic; cook, stirring quickly and frequently for 2 minutes. Add zucchini, pepper and carrots; stir-fry 2-3 minutes or until all vegetables are crisp tender. Stir corn starch mixture and add to skillet. Stir constantly, bring to a boil over medium heat for 1 minute. Stir in tomato, basil and lemon juice; cook for another minute. Makes 6 servings.

Calories: 73
Protein: 4 grams
Carbohydrates: 6 grams

Fat: 0.5 grams
Fiber: 6 grams
Sodium: 183 mg

Asparagus Stir-fry

1 tablespoon cornstarch
3/4 cup reduced-sodium chicken broth
2 tablespoons reduced-sodium soy sauce
3/4 pound fresh asparagus, trimmed
   and cut into 2-inch pieces
1/2 medium green pepper, julienned stips
1/4 cup sliced green onions
1 garlic clove, minced
8 ounces sliced mushrooms
1 can (8 ounces) water chestnuts, drained

In a small bowl, combine cornstarch, broth and soy sauce until smooth; set aside. In a large skillet or wok, stir-fry asparagus, green pepper, onions and garlic in 1 tablespoon hot broth for 2-3 minutes. Add mushrooms; stir-fry for 1-2 minutes. Add water chestnuts; stir-fry 1-2 minutes longer. Stir broth mixture; add to vegetables. Bring to boil; cook and stir for 2 minutes or until thickened. Makes 3 servings.

Calories: 95
Protein: 6 grams
Carbohydrates: 19 grams

Fat: 0.8 grams
Fiber: 4.5 grams
Sodium: 349 mg

Steamed Fresh Vegetables

<u>Large Volume Recipe</u>

1 pound asparagus, 2 inches of stalk
   cut off
1 pound baby carrots
2 pounds broccoli crowns, stalks removed
4 medium zucchini, cut in 2 inch chunks
8 ounces of mushrooms, remove stems

In very large pot, place a steaming basket and 1 inch of water. Wash and prepare vegetables. In order, place carrots, zucchini, broccoli, asparagus and mushrooms in pot. Steam on high heat for 8-10 minutes until asparagus is crisp tender. Serves 8.

Calories: 79   *Fat: 1 gram*
Protein: 6 grams   *Fiber: 6 grams*
Carbohydrates: 16 grams   *Sodium: 48 mg*

Broccoli Mushroom Saute

<u>Quick</u>

5-1/2 cups broccoli florets
1/2 cup thinly sliced green onions
4 garlic cloves, minced
2 tablespoons lemon juice
1/2 teaspoon salt
1/4 teaspoon pepper
8 ounces mushrooms, sliced

In a large pot, bring 1 inch of water to a boil. Place broccoli in a steamer basket over water: cover and steam for 4-5 minutes or until crisp tender. In a skillet coated with nonstick cooking spray, sauté onions over medium heat for 2 minutes. Add garlic and mushrooms and cook for 2 minutes. Add garlic and mushrooms and cook for 2 minutes. Add the broccoli, lemon juice, salt and pepper: toss to coat. Remove from heat and serve. Makes 6 servings.

Calories: 31   *Fat: 0.3 grams*
Protein: 3 grams   *Fiber: 2.6 grams*
Carbohydrates: 6 grams   *Sodium: 214 mg*

SNACKS & APPETIZERS

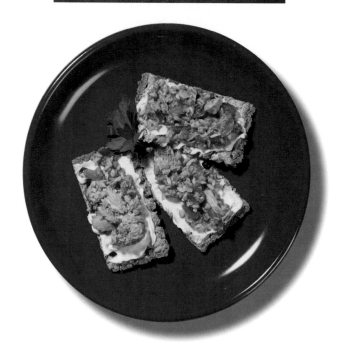

Salmon Crackers

2 fat free rye crisp crackers (15 grams)
1 ounce nonfat cream cheese
1 ounce salmon, canned
1 tablespoon salsa

Mix salsa with salmon. Place half cream cheese then salmon mix on each cracker. 1 serving.

Calories: 116   *Fat: 2 grams*
Protein: 12 grams *Fiber: 4 grams*
Carbohydrates: 12 grams *Sodium: 433 mg*

Cottage Cheese and Yogurt Mix

1/2 cup nonfat cottage cheese
1/2 cup nonfat yogurt (light)

Mix together for a great snack.

Calories: 121   *Fat: 0*
Protein: 19 grams *Fiber: 0*
Carbohydrates: 10 grams *Sodium: 370 mg*

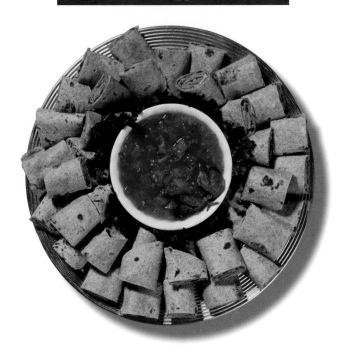

Black Bean Pinwheels

8 ounces of nonfat cream cheese
1 cup nonfat sour cream
1 cup nonfat shredded cheddar cheese
1/4 teaspon garlic powder
15 ounce can black beans, drained
10 whole wheat flour tortillas (10 inch)
Salsa

Blend cream cheese and sour cream in medium bowl. Stir in cheese and garlic powder. Cover; refrigerate for 2 hours. Process beans in food processor until smooth. Spread thin layer beans and thin layer cheese mixture over tortillas. Roll tortillas up tightly. Wrap in plastic wrap and refrigerate until chilled. Cut tortillas crosswise into 7 slices. Serve with salsa. Serves 24; 3 slices each.

Calories: 120   *Fat: 1 grams*
Protein: 9 grams   *Fiber: 2.6 grams*
Carbohydrates: 21 grams *Sodium: 504 mg*

Beans & Salsa Dip

<u>Quick and Large Volume</u>

1 cup salsa
1/2 cup nonfat refried beans
1/2 cup black beans

Mix all ingredients. Serve with baked tortilla chips or vegetables. Serves 8; 4 tablespoons per serving.

Calories: 36 grams   *Fat: 0*
Protein: 2 grams   *Fiber: 2 grams*
Carbohydrates: 6 grams *Sodium: 208 mg*

Chicken Stuffed Potato

<u>Quick</u>

1 medium baking potato (202 grams)
3 ounces cooked chicken breast, chopped
2 tablespoons salsa

Use a fork and pierce potato skin. Bake in microwave for 7-10 minutes or until tender. Slice open and fill with chicken. Top with salsa. Serves 1.

Calories: 368   *Fat: 3 grams*
Protein: 31 grams   *Fiber: 5 grams*
Carbohydrates: 52 grams *Sodium: 631 mg*

Baked Potato topped with Cottage Cheese

<u>Quick</u>

1 medium baking potato (202 grams)
1 cup nonfat cottage cheese
Salsa (optional)

Use a fork and pierce potato skin. Bake in microwave for 7-10 minutes or until tender. Slice open and fill with cottage cheese. Top with salsa. Serves 1.

Calories: 342   *Fat: 0 grams*
Protein: 29 grams   *Fiber: 5 grams*
Carbohydrates: 54 grams *Sodium: 597 mg*

Cowboy Caviar *by Jan Lutz*

<u>Quick and Large Volume</u>

Great for BBQ's or Potlucks!

2-15 ounce cans black beans, rinsed
   and drained
1-10 ounce bag frozen white corn,
   defrosted
1 pint cherry tomatoes, diced
1 medium red onion, diced
1/2 bunch cilantro, chopped
2 ripe avocados, diced

Mix it up! Makes 20 servings.

Calories: 110	Fat: 3.5 grams
Protein: 5 grams	Fiber: 5.5 grams
Carbohydrates: 17 grams	Sodium: 105 mg

Tuna Spread for Whatever *by Nancy VanHoven*

<u>Quick</u>

6 ounces Albacore tuna, drained
6 egg whites, cooked
1 tablespoon chopped green onion
2 tablespoons chopped celery
1/4 cup 1000 island dressing, fat-free

Mix all ingredients. Serve on rye crackers,
pita bread, stuff tomatoes, use as a
vegetable dip or whatever! Serves 4.

Calories: 97	Fat: 0.7 grams
Protein: 16 grams	Fiber: 0 grams
Carbohydrates: 7 grams	Sodium: 480 mg

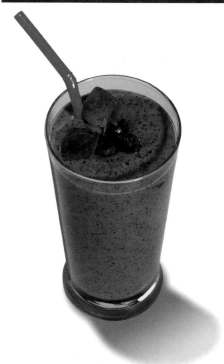

Blueberry-Peach Smoothie

<u>Quick</u>

1 cup nonfat vanilla yogurt
1 cup fresh blueberries halves
1 medium peach
Ice

Blend all ingredients and add a few ice cubes at a time. Add ice until shake is desired consistency. Serves 1.

Calories: 208   *Fat: 0.6 gram*
Protein: 15 grams   *Fiber: 5 grams*
Carbohydrates: 39   *Sodium: 161 mg*

Banana-Strawberry Smoothie

<u>Quick</u>

1 cup nonfat vanilla yogurt
1 cup fresh strawberry halves
1 medium banana
1/4 cup apple juice
Ice

Blend all ingredients and add a few ice cubes at a time. Add ice until shake is desired consistency. Serves 1.

Calories: 274   *Fat: 1 gram*
Protein: 15 grams   *Fiber: 7 grams*
Carbohydrates: 56 grams *Sodium: 163 mg*

DESSERTS & SWEETS

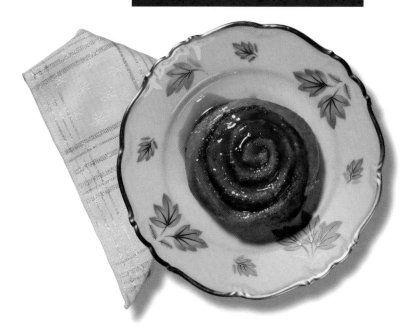

Fat-Free Cinnamon Rolls

<u>Large Volume</u>

3/4 cup nonfat milk
1/2 cup sugar
1 teaspoon salt
1/2 cup applesauce
2 packets active dry yeast
1/3 cup warm water
    (105-115 degrees F)
3/4 cup egg substitute
1-1/2 cup powdered sugar
2-1/2 cups whole wheat flour
2-1/2 cups flour

Filling:

Light margarine cinnamon,
    brown sugar, sugar

Glaze topping:

1/3 cup evaporated skim milk
2 tablespoon brown sugar
1-1/2 cup powdered sugar
1 teaspoon vanilla extract

Combine milk, sugar, salt, and applesauce in bowl. Microwave for 1-2 minutes until sugar dissolves. Cool to lukewarm. Dissolve yeast in warm water. Add milk mixture, eggs, and 2 cups each of flours. Attach dough hook to mixer. Turn to low-medium speed for 2 minutes or mix by hand by kneading. Continue on low-medium speed, add remaining flour, 1/2 cup at a time, until dough clings to hook and side of the bowl, about 2 minutes. Continue kneading another 2 minutes. Place in greased bowl, turning to grease top. Cover; let rise in warm place, free from draft, until double in bulk, about 1 hour. Punch down dough. Place on floured surface and roll out to 1/4 inch. Spread light margarine lightly over surface. Sprinkle with brown sugar, cinnamon, and very lightly with sugar. Roll dough from long side. Cut into 21 rolls and place on cookie sheet. Let rise for 45-60 minutes. Bake for 15-18 minutes at 350 degrees. For glaze, heat milk and brown sugar in microwave for 1 minute or until brown sugar dissolves. Whip in powdered sugar and vanilla until creamy. Pour over cooled rolls. Serves 21.

Calories: 201   *Fat: 0.5 grams*
Protein: 5 grams   *Fiber: 2 grams*
Carbohydrates: 45 grams   *Sodium: 160 mg*

Maple Bars

Use the cinnamon roll dough following the same directions up until rolling out the dough. Instead place on floured surface and roll out to about 1 inch thick. Cut into 16 rectangles. Place on cookie sheet and let rise for 40 minutes. Bake at 350 degrees for 15-22 minutes or until lightly brown. Serves 16.

Maple Glaze - Same as cinnamon roll glaze topping except add 1/2 teaspoon maple extract.

Calories: 250
Protein: 7 grams
Carbohydrates: 53 grams
Fat: 0.6 grams
Fiber: 2.6 grams
Sodium: 200 mg

Whole Wheat Banana Bread

1 cup flour
3/4 cup whole wheat flour
1 teaspoon baking soda
1/4 teaspoon salt
1/2 cup sugar
3/4 cup applesauce
1/4 cup egg substitute
2 ripe bananas
1 teaspoon pure vanilla extract

Preheat oven to 350 degrees. Mix all dry ingredients in medium bowl. Beat all other ingredients in large bowl. Add flour mixture slowly and mix well. Pour into loaf pan sprayed with cooking spray. Bake for 40-45 minutes. Serves 12.

Calories: 123
Protein: 3 grams
Carbohydrates: 28 grams
Fat: 0.3 grams
Fiber: 2 grams
Sodium: 161 mg

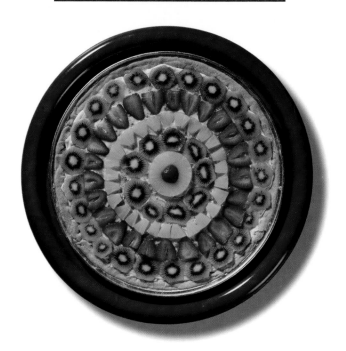

Fruit Pizza

<u>Large Volume</u>

1 roll sugar cookie dough (18 ounce roll)
1/2 cup whole wheat flour
1 block nonfat cream cheese
1 cup powdered sugar
1/4 teaspoon almond extract
1/2 cup apricot jam
3 large kiwis sliced
2 cup sliced strawberries
1 small can pineapple chunks

Preheat oven to 350 degrees. Roll out cookie dough on whole wheat floured surface. Make a large round (16 inch) circle with dough. Bake on cookie sheet for 15 minutes. Let cool. Mix cream cheese and powdered sugar and almond extract until creamy. Spread cream cheese mix over baked cookie crust. On top of cream cheese mixture, spread the apricot jam to make a thin layer. Arrange fruit on pizza as you like. Refrigerate for 1-2 hours. Serves 16.

Calories: 235   *Fat: 7 grams*
Protein: 8 grams   *Fiber: 2 grams*
Carbohydrates: 35 grams *Sodium: 371 mg*

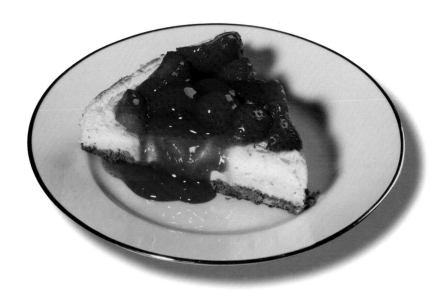

Low-fat Creamy Cheesecake

3-8 ounce nonfat cream cheese blocks
16 ounces nonfat sour cream
1/2 cup egg substitute
3/4 cup sugar (or sugar substitute)
3/4 teaspoon salt (optional)
1/4 teaspoon ground ginger
2 teaspoon pure vanilla extract
10 low-fat graham crackers

Cheesecake Toppings

Add your favorite fruit such as sliced strawberries, raspberries, blueberries or cooked apples.

Preheat oven to 350 degrees. Crush graham crackers and line bottom of cheesecake pan. Whip cream cheese until smooth. Add sour cream and blend until smooth. Add the remaining ingredients except for the crackers. Pour mixture over crushed graham crackers in pan. Bake for 52-60 minutes. Chill for at least 2 hours or overnight. Serves 8.

Calories: 241   *Fat: 2 grams*
Protein: 16 grams   *Fiber: 1 gram*
Carbohydrates: 38 grams   *Sodium: 600 mg*

Banana Cream Dessert

2-(2.1 ounce) packages fat free, sugar free
   vanilla pudding
2-3/4 cup nonfat milk
1/4 cup fat free vanilla coffee creamer
1 medium banana
10 low-fat graham crackers, crushed
Cool-whip Free (nonfat dairy topping)

Prepare pudding mix as directed on package except only add 2-3/4 cup milk and 1/4 cup vanilla coffee creamer. Place graham cracker crumbs in a glass 9" pie pan and spread evenly. Slice 1/2 of the banana on top of the cracker crumbs. Pour pudding mix over bananas. Slice the other 1/2 of banana on top. Top with cool whip and refrigerate for 2 hours. Serves 8.

Calories: 203   *Fat: 3.5 grams*
Protein: 5 grams   *Fiber: 1 gram*
Carbohydrates: 37 grams   *Sodium: 831 mg*

Oatmeal Raisin Cookies

<u>Large Volume</u>

1 cup unsweetened applesauce
3/4 cup brown sugar
1/2 cup sugar (or sugar substitute)
4 egg whites
1 teaspoon pure vanilla extract
3/4 cup flour
3/4 cup whole wheat flour
1 teaspoon baking soda
1 teaspoon cinnamon
1/2 teaspoon salt (optional)
3 cups old fashioned oats, uncooked
1 cup raisins
1/2 cup vanilla protein powder

Preheat oven to 350 degrees. Beat applesauce and sugar together. Add egg whites and vanilla; beat well. In separate bowl, combine flours, soda, cinnamon, salt and protein powder. Add slowly to applesauce mixture until blended. Add oats and raisins. Drop by teaspoons on baking sheet and bake for 14 minutes. Cool and place on wire rack. Makes 3 dozen.

Calories: 83   *Fat: 0.2 grams*
Protein: 2 grams   *Fiber: 2 grams*
Carbohydrates: 19 grams   *Sodium: 46 mg*

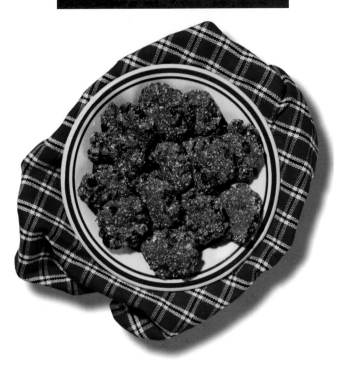

Sugar-free Oatmeal Cookies *by Cindy Marshall*

1 cup light vanilla yogurt
1/2 cup sugar substitute
1 small package sugar-free banana
   instant pudding mix
4 egg whites
1/4 cup nonfat milk
2 teaspoons vanilla
1-1/4 cup whole wheat flour
1 teaspoon baking soda
1 teaspoon salt
2-1/2 cups oatmeal, dry
1 cup raisins
1 teaspoon cinnamon
1 teaspoon nutmeg
1/3 cup chopped pecans

Mix dry ingredients. Add in all other ingredients. Mix well. Spoon onto cookie sheet coated with cooking spray. Press slightly to flaten. Bake at 350 degrees for 10-12 minutes. Makes 2 dozen.

Calories: 90   *Fat: 1.5 grams*
Protein: 3 grams   *Fiber: 2 grams*
Carbohydrates: 17 grams *Sodium: 130 mg*

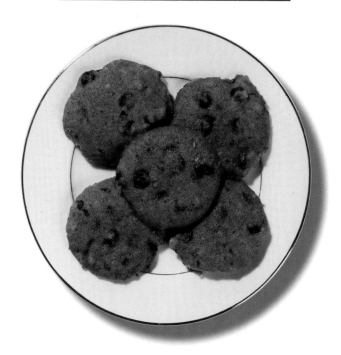

Whole Wheat Chocolate Chip Cookies

1-1/4 cup flour
1 cup whole wheat flour
1 teaspoon baking soda
3/4 teaspoon salt (optional)
1 cup unsweetened applesauce
3/4 cup sugar
3/4 cup brown sugar
1 teaspoon vanilla
4 egg whites
1 cup semi sweet chocolate chips
1/2 cup chopped walnuts (optional)

Preheat oven to 375 degrees. Combine flours, soda, and salt in small bowl. Beat applesauce, sugars, and vanilla in large mixing bowl. Add egg whites and beat well. Gradually, add flour mixture. Stir in chocolate chips and nuts. Drop by teaspoons onto baking sheet. Bake for 10-13 minutes or until golden brown. Makes 4 dozen cookies.

Calories: 75   *Fat: 2 grams*
Protein: 1 gram   *Fiber: 1 gram*
Carbohydrates: 14 grams Sodium: 69 mg

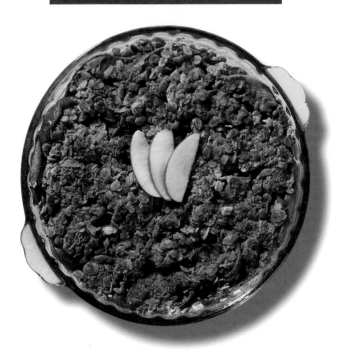

Mock Apple Pie

7 cooking apples (Golden, Rome, Granny)
3/4 cup old fashioned regular oatmeal
   (uncooked)
1/2 cup vanilla protein powder
1 cup sugar substitute
1 tablespoon cinnamon
1 tablespoon whole wheat flour
1/2 cup apple juice

Heat oven to 350 degrees. Spray 9 inch pie pan with non-stick spray. Sprinkle 1/4 cup oatmeal in bottom. In large mixing bowl, slice or shred apple (cored) with peel. Add sugar substitute, cinnamon, apple juice and flour. Pour into pan. Mix other 1/2 cup oatmeal and protein powder. Pour over apples. Spray topping with cooking spray for moisture. Bake for 35 minutes uncovered, and then cover with foil for 10 more minutes. Serve with nonfat whipped topping. Serves 12.

Calories: 153   *Fat: 2 grams*
Protein: 5 grams   *Fiber 5 grams*
Carbohydrates: 31 grams   *Sodium: 82 mg*

Baked Apple

1 baking apple (Golden Delicious, Jonathan)
1/2 teaspoon sugar substitute
1 tablespoon apple juice
1/2 teaspoon cinnamon

Remove the stem and core of apples. Place in a shallow glass baking dish. Pour apple juice over apple, sprinkle with sugar substitute and cinnamon. Bake, uncovered, in preheated oven 350 degrees for 45 minutes. Or, cover with plastic wrap and microwave for 7-10 minutes or until apple is tender. Makes 1 serving.

Calories: 82   *Fat: 0.5 grams*
Protein: 1 gram   *Fiber 5 grams*
Carbohydrates: 21 grams   *Sodium: 3 mg*

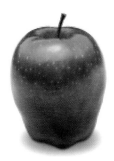

Red Delicious

Deep ruby skin and a classic heart shape. Its mild, sweet flavor and juicy crunch make it one of America's most popular snacking apples

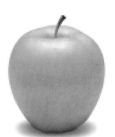

Golden Delicious

The preferred all-purpose cooking apple. Firm, white flesh and skin so tender it doesn't require peeling. Maintains its shape and rich, mellow flavor after cooking.

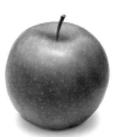

Granny Smith

Bright green, sometimes with a pink blush. Tart tangy flavor and crisp bite. Great for cooking or a take along snack.

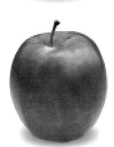

Pink Lady™

Delicious sweet-tart taste and firm, crisp flesh. Pink Lady is yellow in color with a pink blush. Great apple for cooking or eating out of hand.

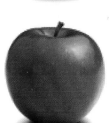

Rome Beauty

The bright red Rome Beauty is used primarily for cooking because the flavor grows richer when baked or sautéd. Often referred to as the "baker's buddy."

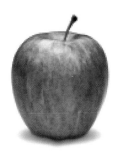

Gala

Heartshaped, distinctive yellow-orange skin with red striping and a crisp, sweet taste. Great in salads or eating out of hand.

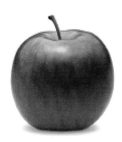

Fuji

The Fuji varies from yellow-green with red highlights to very red. Crisp and juicy with a spicy, sweet flavor. Excellent in salads or eating out of hand.

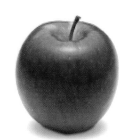

Braeburn

Varying from greenish-gold with red sections to nearly solid red, the crisp, aromatic Braeburn's blend of sweetness and tartness delivers high impact flavor. Great for snacks or salads.

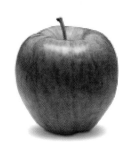

Cameo™

The Cameo offers rich sweet taste and firm-texture. Its color is red stripe over a creamy background. Excellent for desserts or snacking.

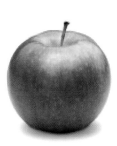

Jonagold

A blend of Jonathan and Golden Delicious. Yellow-green base with a blush stripe. Unique tangy-sweet flavor. Great for cooking or just plain eating.

References

1. Davy Brenda M., Melby Christopher L. *The effect of fiber-rich carbohydrates on features of Syndrome X*. J Am Diet Assoc 2003;103:86-96.

2. Mayo Clinic. *Special Report: Weight Control*. Supplement to Foundation for Medical Education and Research Publications 2003.

3. American Dietetic Association. *Dietary Reference Intakes Released For Carbohydrates, Fats, Protein, Fiber and Physical Activity*. Fall 2002;volume 2.

4. Jenkins DJ, Wolever TM, Vuksan V et al. *Nibbling versus gorging: metabolic advantages of increased meal frequency*. New Eng J Med 1989;321:929-934.

5. Jequier E. *Response to and range of acceptable fat intake in adults*. Eur J Clin Nutr. 1999 Apr;53:S84-93.

6. Simopoulos AP. *Essential fatty acids in health and chronic disease*. Am J Clin Nutr 1999 Sep;70:560S-569S.

7. Rolls B. *The role of energy density in the overconsumption of fat*. J Nutr 2000;130:268S-271S.

8. Rolls B, Bell EA, Castellanos VH et al. *Energy density but not fat content of foods affected energy intake in lean and obese women*. Am J Clin Nutr 1999 May;69:863-871.

9. Levine AS, Billington CJ. *Dietary fiber: does it affect food intake and body weight?* In: Fernstrom substitutes. Boca Raton, FL:CRC Press, 1994:191-200.

10. American Heart Assoc. *Media Advisory: American Heart Associations Statement on High-Protein, Low-Carbohydrate Diet Study Presented at Scientific Sessions*. Nov 2002.

11. Layman DK, Shiue H, Sather C et al. *Increased dietary protein modifies glucose and insulin homeostasis in adult women during weight loss*. J Nutr 2003;133:405-410.

12. Layman DK, Boileau RA, Erickson D et al. *A reduced ratio of dietary carbohydrates to protein improves body composition and blood lipid*

profiles during weight loss in adult women. J Nutr 2003;133(2):411-417.

13. Conceicao de Oliveira M, Sichieri R, Moura AS. *Weight loss associated with a daily intake of three apples or three pears among overweight women.* Nutr 2003;19:253-256.

14. Howarth NC, Saltzman E, Roberts SB. *Dietary fiber and weight regulation.* Nutr Rev 2001;59(5):129.

15. Golay A, Eigenheer C, Morel Y et al. *Weight loss with low or high carbohydrate diet?* Int J Obes Relat Metab Disord 1996;20:1067.

16. Frost G, Lees A, Dore' CJ, et al. *Glycemic index as a determinant of serum HDL-cholesterol concentration.* Lancet 1999;353:1045.

17. Katan MB. *Are there good and bad carbohydrates for HDL cholesterol?* Lancet 1999;353:1029.

18. Foster-Powell K, Miller JB. *International tables of glycemic index.* Am J Clin Nutr 1995;62:871S.

19. Bessesen DH. *The role of carbohydrates in insulin resistance.* J Nutr 2001;131:2782S.

20. Roberts SB. *High-glycemic index foods, hunger, and obesity: is there a connection?* Nutr Rev 2000;58:163.

21. Keim NL, Van Loan MD, Horn WF et al. *Weight loss is greater with consumption of large morning meals and fat-free mass is preserved with large evening meals in women on a controlled weight reduction regimen.* J Nutr 1997;127:75-82.

22. Barzel US, Massey LK. *Excess dietary protein can adversely affect bone.* J Nutr 1998;128:1051-1053.

23. Heshka S, Yang MU, Wang J et al. *Weight loss and changes in resting metabolic rate.* Am J Clin Nutr 1990;52:981-986.

24. Kelsay JL, Behall KM, Prather ES. *Effect of fiber from fruits and vegetables on metabolic responses of human subjects I. Bowel transit time, number of defecations, fecal weight, urinary excretions of energy and nitrogen and apparent digestibilities of energy, nitrogen, and fat.* Am J Clin Nutr 1978;31:1149-1153.

25. Raben A, Christensen NJ, Madsen J et al. *Decreased postprandial thermogenesis and fat oxidation but increased fullness after a high-fiber meal compared with a low-fiber meal.* Am J Clin Nutr 1994;59:1386-1394.

26. Wing RR, Hill JO. *Successful weight loss maintenance.* Annu Rev Nutr 2001;21:323-341.

27. Hill JO, Melanson EL, Wyatt HT. *Dietary fat intake and regulation of energy balance: Implications for obesity.* J Nutr 2000;130:284S-288S.

28. Klem ML, Wing RR, McGuire MT et al. *A descriptive study of individuals successful at long-term maintenance of substantial weight loss.* Am J Clin Nutr 1997;66:239-246.

29. Freese R, Alfthan G, Jauhiainen M et al. *High intakes of vegetables, berries, and apples combined with a high intake of linoleic or oleic acid only slightly affect markers of lipid peroxidation and lipoprotein metabolism in healthy subjects.* Am J Clin Nutr 2002;76:950-960.

30. Lampe JA. *Health effects of vegetables and fruit: assessing mechanisms of action in human experimental studies.* Am J Clin Nutr 1999;70:475S-490S.

31. Moore MC, Cherrington AD, Mann SL et al. *Acute fructose administration decreases the glycemic response to an oral glucose tolerance test in normal adults.* Clin Endocrinol Metab 2000;85:4515.

32. McCrory MA, Fuss PJ, Saltzman E et al. *Dietary determinants of energy intake and weight regulation in healthy adults.* J Nutr 2000;130:276S.

33. Brand-Miller J, Wolever T, Colagiuri S, Foster-Powell K. *The Glucose Revolution.* Marlowe & Company, New York 1999.

34. Simopoulos AP, Robinson J. *The Omega Diet.* Harper Perennial, New York 1999.

35. Clark N. *Sports Nutrition Guidebook.* Human Kinetics, IL 1997.

36. DesMaisons K. *Potatoes not Prozac.* Simon & Schuster, New York 1998.

37. Insel P, Turner RE, Ross D. *Nutrition.* Jones and Bartlett Publishers, Mass 2001.

38. Evans W, Rosenberg I. *BioMarkers.* Simon & Schuster, New York 1992.

39. Muldoon MF, Kritchevsky SB. *Flavonoid intake and coronary mortality in Finland: a cohort study.* British Medical Journal 1996;312:478-481.

40. Hyson D, Studebarker-Hallman D, Davis PA et al. *Apple juice consumption reduces plasma Low-Density Lipoprotein oxidation in healthy men and women.* Journal of Medicinal Food 2000;3:159-165.

41. Brand-Miller J, Wolever T, Colagiuri S, Foster-Powell K. *The New Glucose Revolution*. Marlowe & Company, New York 2003.

42. Katz D. *The Way to Eat.* Sourcebooks, Illinois 2002.

Other resources and recommended reading

American Dietetic Association	www.eatright.org
American Academy of Family Physicians	www.aafp.org
American Medical Association	www.ama-assn.org
American Diabetes Association	www.diabetics.org
Centers for Disease Control	www.cdc.gov
Department of Agriculture:	
Food and Nutrition Information Center	www.nal.usda.gov/fnic
Weight Control Information Network	

www.niddk.nih.gov/health/nutrit/win.htm

Body for Life by Bill Phillips
Sports Nutrition Guidebook by Nancy Clark M.S, R.D.
Food Values of Portions Commonly Used by Jean A.T. Pennington.
The NutriBase Complete Book of Food Counts
Women's health & Wellness 2003 Real life solutions
    from the editors of *Health* magazine
Better Homes and Gardens, *New Cook Book*
Taste of Homes *Light and Tasty* magazine
Eating Well, The magazine of food & health
Food Works Nutrition Analysis Software

FOOD AND BEVERAGE RECORD

Date from_____ to_____   Blood Pressure_____

Day_____

Time	Food & beverage quantity	Kcals*	Pro (g)	Carb (g)	Fat (g)	Fiber (g)
	Totals					

Kcals = calories   (g) = grams

Begin each exercise session with a five minute warm-up and stretch. Warming up includes walking in place or using your favorite cardio equipment, stepping, jumping jacks, twisting and arm circles. Follow your warm-up with light stretching. Rest between sets should be 60-90 seconds. The progression you have here assumes someone who has had little exercise experience.

This is just one idea for a simple 3-day-a-week plan. The number of sets for you to do is listed before the number of repetitions for that set (2 sets x 12 repetitions).

Repetitions
(called reps)

This refers to the number of times you actually move the weight through its full range of motion. You lift your child from the ground to overhead 10 times in a row before resting and you have performed 10 repetitions of "child presses"! Your repetitions are increased as the weeks go by. You will also be increasing the amount of weight that you use. If you can complete your sets and repetitions with good form, increase your weight on your next workout by about 5%.

Sets

A set is a group of repetitions. You would normally rest after each set. It is recommended that you rest for only 60-90 seconds.

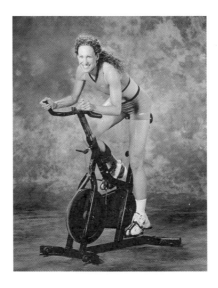

12-WEEK BEGINNER'S EXERCISE PROGRAM

Weeks, Sets and Repetitions

Day & Exercise		Weeks 1-2	Weeks 3-4	Weeks 5-6	Weeks 7-8	Weeks 9-10	Weeks 11-12
Monday	Squats	1x8	2x8	2x10	3x12	3x12	3x15
	Lunges	1x8	2x8	2x10	3x12	3x12	3x15
	Dumbbell Chest Press	1x8	2x8	2x10	3x12	3x12	3x15
	Triceps Pushdowns	1x8	2x8	2x10	3x12	3x12	3x15
	Ab*-crunches	1x20	2x20	2x25	3x25	3x30	3x30
	Cardiovascular**	15 min	20 min	25 min	30 min	35 min	35 min
	Stretch	5 min	5 min	5 min	5 min	5 min	5 min
Tuesday	Cardiovascular**	15 min	20 min	30 min	30 min	40 min	40 min
	Stretch	5 min	5 min	5 min	5 min	5 min	5 min
Wednesday	Leg Press	1x8	2x8	2x10	3x12	3x12	3x15
	Leg Curls	1x8	2x8	2x10	3x12	3x12	3x15
	Lat Pull-downs	1x8	2x8	2x10	3x12	3x12	3x15
	Dumbbell Bicep Curls	1x8	2x8	2x10	3x12	3x12	3x15
	Reverse Crunch (Abs)	1x20	2x20	2x25	3x25	3x30	3x30
	Cardiovascular**	15 min	20 min	25 min	30 min	35 min	35 min
	Stretch	5 min	5 min	5 min	5 min	5 min	5 min
Thursday	Cardiovascular**	15 min	20 min	30 min	30 min	40 min	40 min
	Stretch	5 min	5 min	5 min	5 min	5 min	5 min
Friday	Squats	11x8	2x8	2x10	3x12	3x12	3x15
	Lunges	1x8	2x8	2x10	3x12	3x12	3x15
	Overhead Press	1x8	2x8	2x10	3x12	3x12	3x15
	Push-ups	1x8	2x8	2x10	3x12	3x12	3x15
	Ab*-crunches	1x20	2x20	2x25	3x25	3x30	3x30
	Cardiovascular**	15 min	20 min	25 min	30 min	35 min	35 min
	Stretch	5 min	5 min	5 min	5 min	5 min	5 min
Saturday & Sunday	Cardiovascular**	15 min	20 min	25 min	30 min	35 min	35 min
	Stretch	5 min	5 min	5 min	5 min	5 min	5 min

*Ab (Abdominal) crunches
**Cardiovascular training can be walking, cycling, running, jumping jacks or rope, stair climbing, exercise videos or other cardiovascular exercise machines at the gym.

Ask a trainer for proper demonstration of exercises or other exercise programs. You may get different recommendations from a trainer. That's okay, trainers have good reasons for their recommendations!

WEEKLY EXERCISE TRACKING

Week #_____

Day/Date	Cardiovascular	Intensity/Heart Rate* Duration/Mins.	Weight Training	Comments
Monday _____	__Treadmill __Bike __Stair Step __Aerobic Class _____Other	__80-100 __110-130 __10-20 __25-35 __140-160 __160-180 __40-60 __60-90	__Upper body __Lower Body __Overall Body __Sculpt/Group class	
Tuesday _____	__Treadmill __Bike __Stair Step __Aerobic Class _____Other	__80-100 __110-130 __10-20 __25-35 __140-160 __160-180 __40-60 __60-90	__Upper body __Lower Body __Overall Body __Sculpt/Group class	
Wednesday _____	__Treadmill __Bike __Stair Step __Aerobic Class _____Other	__80-100 __110-130 __10-20 __25-35 __140-160 __160-180 __40-60 __60-90	__Upper body __Lower Body __Overall Body __Sculpt/Group class	
Thursday _____	__Treadmill __Bike __Stair Step __Aerobic Class _____Other	__80-100 __110-130 __10-20 __25-35 __140-160 __160-180 __40-60 __60-90	__Upper body __Lower Body __Overall Body __Sculpt/Group class	
Friday _____	__Treadmill __Bike __Stair Step __Aerobic Class _____Other	__80-100 __110-130 __10-20 __25-35 __140-160 __160-180 __40-60 __60-90	__Upper body __Lower Body __Overall Body __Sculpt/Group class	
Saturday _____	__Treadmill __Bike __Stair Step __Aerobic Class _____Other	__80-100 __110-130 __10-20 __25-35 __140-160 __160-180 __40-60 __60-90	__Upper body __Lower Body __Overall Body __Sculpt/Group class	
Sunday _____	__Treadmill __Bike __Stair Step __Aerobic Class _____Other	__80-100 __110-130 __10-20 __25-35 __140-160 __160-180 __40-60 __60-90	__Upper body __Lower Body __Overall Body __Sculpt/Group class	
Sample 1/15/03	__Treadmill _x_Bike __Stair Step __Aerobic Class _____Other	__80-100 __110-130 __10-20 __25-35 _x_140-160 __160-180 _x_40-60 __60-90	__Upper body __Lower Body _x_Overall Body __Sculpt/Group class	Exercise felt great today!

* To find your heart rate, wear a heart rate monitor or check your pulse on the wrist or neck. Count the beats in six seconds. Then multiply the number by 10. For example: The number after six seconds is 13. 13x10=130 beats per minute.

Target heart rate calculation: 220-age= Maximum heart rate. Take your maximum heart rate and times it by 65%-85%= target heart rate. Example: 220-36=184. 184x.65=120 beats per minute.

Recipe Index

Breakfast Foods

Protein Foods

Eggs

Shakes

Chicken, Turkey, Fish & Beef

Combinations

Main Entrees

Salads and Vegetables

Snacks and Appetizers

Desserts and Sweets

Apple Varieties

Index

Place "before" photo here.

- FRONT -

Place "before" photo here.

- BACK -

After Photos

Place "after" photo here.

- FRONT -

Place "after" photo here.

- BACK -

Before Photos

Place "before" photo here.

- FRONT -

Place "before" photo here.

- BACK -

After Photos

Place *"after"* photo here.

- FRONT -

Place *"after"* photo here.

- BACK -

Favorite Recipes

Favorite Recipes

Favorite Recipes

Favorite Recipes

Favorite Recipes

Favorite Recipes

Favorite Recipes

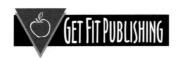

Quick Order Form

Fax Orders: 509-888-5329

Email Orders: www.3appleplan.com

Postal Orders: Get Fit Publishing

P.O. Box 2226

Wenatchee, WA 98807-2226 USA

Please send:

❏ A copy of this book, **The "3 Apple-a-Day" Plan** for $29.95 + $5.00
shipping and handling to:

❏ **The Total Success Kit**™—a 12-week, 20-page, full-color guide featuring
the "3 Apple-a-Day" Plan for $9.95 + $1.00 shipping and handling to:

Name:_____

Address:_____

City:_____State:____Zip:_____

Telephone:_____

Email address:_____

Sales tax: Please add 8% to Washington state addresses.

Product $ _____ x _____ quantity = $ _____

Product $ _____ x _____ quantity = $ _____

Shipping $ _____

Tax $ _____

Total $ _____

Payment:

❏ Check

❏ Credit card: Visa   Mastercard   AMEX   Discover

Card number:_____

Name on card:_____Exp. Date:_____